# CLINICAL RESEARCH ISSUES IN NURSING

# NURSING - ISSUES, PROBLEMS AND CHALLENGES

Additional books in this series can be found on Nova's website under the Series tab.

Additional E-books in this series can be found on Nova's website under the E-book tab.

# CLINICAL RESEARCH ISSUES IN NURSING

## ZENOBIA C.Y. CHAN
### EDITOR

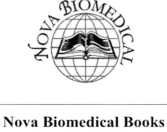

Nova Biomedical Books
*New York*

## Library of Congress Cataloging-in-Publication Data

Chan, Zenobia C. Y.
  Clinical research issues in nursing / Zenobia C.Y. Chan.
      p. ; cm.
  Includes bibliographical references and index.
  ISBN 978-1-61668-937-7 (hardcover)
  1. Nursing--Research. 2. Nursing--Abstracting and indexing. I. Title.
  [DNLM: 1. Clinical Nursing Research. 2. Abstracting and Indexing as
Topic. 3. Ethics, Research. 4. Periodicals as Topic. 5. Research Design.
6. Writing. WY 20.5 C433c 2010]
  RT81.5.C43 2010
  610.73072--dc22
                          2010025435

*Published by Nova Science Publishers, Inc.* † *New York*

# Contents

# Preface

There are few Asian nurse researchers, especially in Hong Kong, who have written about issues related to clinical research in nursing. Little has been mentioned in previous literature regarding clinical research issues in nursing such as the art of abstract writing in academic journals, the strategies of literature review, critical analysis of various research designs and approaches such as ethnography, grounded theory, experimental designs, surveys, structured interviews, observation methods, and ethical issues of clinical studies with the collection effort from the master students' contributions. This book is a collection of master nursing students' work that demonstrates the needs and importance of addressing many underexplored issues in clinical issues in nursing. The objectives of this book are: to heighten research students' awareness of the scholarship of both the formulation of research design and the issues of clinical research, and to equip them with ideas and the strategies to develop their own research proposals and implement a research project. This book hopes to offer some contextual understanding on clinical research issues in nursing in a Chinese context.

In: Clinical Research Issues in Nursing     ISBN: 978-1-61668-937-7
Editor: Z. C. Y. Chan, pp.1-11     © 2010 Nova Science Publishers, Inc.

*Chapter I*

# Ways to Write Abstracts Contributing to Publication in Nursing Journals

*F. Hung*[*] *and*
*Zenobia C. Y. Chan*
The Hong Kong Polytechnic University, China

## Abstract

**Background:** Abstract is usually the first part of a research article. It structures the outline and lists the important results and arguments of the study. It is probably the only part that the reader would go through and thus should be concise and directive.

**Objective:** To illustrate the writing style and format of abstract writing in nursing research articles through introducing the types and structures of abstracts and comparing the publishing guidelines of two nursing research journals.

**Discussion:** Informative abstract is commonly used in medical and nursing research because readers can go through the main arguments of the article quickly. The requirement of abstract in *Nursing Research* and *Clinical Nursing Research* are similar. Informative abstract is preferred

---

[*] Correspondence concerning this article should be addressed to: F. Hung, Email: ube725@gmail.com

and word limits are set. Nursing Research requires the use of Medical Subject Headings (MeSH).

**Conclusion:** While keeping the word count to the minimum, a good abstract can present the maximum amount of important arguments, results and implications. In clinical nursing research, having a well-written abstract makes an article stand out and can lead ultimately to publication in academic journals.

**Implication:** Many local medical and nursing journals lack writing guidelines for authors. Good quality journals, like the two discussed, have good control of their contents. Local journals should follow as this is fundamental to academic excellence.

# Introduction

In whichever subject or profession, almost every scholarly written research article includes an abstract, which serves the purpose of listing the important points and results derived from the studies conducted. It also serves the purpose of attracting the potential readers or journal reviewers to go through the complete study paper (Costa-Pierce, 1997; University of California Berkeley, 2003; UNC-CH Writing Center, 2007).

What exactly is an abstract? A number of universities give similar descriptions. For example, University of California Berkeley suggests that abstracts are short summaries of the completed research (University of California Berkeley, 2003); University of North Carolina suggests that abstract is self-contained, short, and powerful and describes a larger work (UNC-CH Writing Center, 2007). Because the term "abstract" has long been a very well-known term in the academic field, Philip Koopman from the Carnegie Mellon University start his guide of writing abstract straightly by introducing its importance (Koopman, 1997). John Cole from the Intel, one of the biggest semiconductor corporation, suggests that abstract is "a brief, written explanation of the research project, consisting of a succinct description of the project's purpose, the procedures followed, the data collected, and the conclusions reached" (Cole, 2008).

Nursing is both a science and an art. The International Council of Nurses believes that research is a hallmark of professional nursing and can generate new knowledge, advance nursing science, evaluate existing practice and services, and provide evidence for nursing education, practice, research and management (International Council of Nurses, 2007). To date, thanks to the advancement of the internet and information technology, there are millions of nursing research articles shared through the internet. There is an overwhelming amount of information and so, the question comes. How can nursing scholars search among these research articles and pick up the most suitable ones for their subsequent work? Abstract can do the trick. With a well-written abstract, communication between readers and research articles can be efficient and effective. Well-written abstract is directive and allows readers to go through the main arguments of the research paper without having to spend too much time. Abstract is one of the deciding factors for the worthiness of the research article (Fisher, 2005). Provided that the study itself was in good quality, a good piece of abstract definitely helps readers to sniff out such good quality research work.

Other than publication in journals, abstracts are required in conferences or symposiums. Good abstracts can attract attention of the organizing bodies (Cole & Koziol-McLain, 1997). Thus, writing up good abstracts is a cornerstone for scholarship and publications.

# Objectives

This article highlights what elements a good abstract should encompass. By comparing and contrasting the guidelines of two internationally renowned nursing journals, the requirements and quality of the abstracts publishing in nursing journals are discussed. More importantly, it is hoped that some insights would be brought to the local academia. Local journals should learn from these internationally renowned journals and establish clear writing guidelines for authors.

# Preparing an Abstract

Guideline from the International Committee of Medical Journal Editors (2009) stated that abstracts should emphasize the new and important aspects of the study. However, it could be very difficult to achieve this goal since condense and concise languages are expected, while still expressing the most amount of important and attractive arguments. This section goes through the ways to achieve the purpose by introducing the two types of abstracts, descriptive and informative abstract (Killborn, 1998; UNC-CH Writing

Center, 2007). More effort is used in discussing the informative abstract, which is more widely used in clinical nursing research.

## Descriptive Abstracts

Descriptive abstracts are usually short (about 100 words) and are considered to be an outline of the article (Killborn, 1998; UNC-CH Writing Center, 2007). No judging statement from the project is included in the abstract. The reader must go through the article in order to learn about the project (Killborn, 1998; UNC-CH Writing Center, 2007). For this reason, descriptive abstracts are getting less popular in academic writing (Colorado State University, 2009).

## Informative Abstracts

Informative abstracts are more than only an outline. Authors would include purpose of study, main arguments, research methods and findings, conclusion and recommendations in the abstract. Thus, when readers go through the abstract, the whole picture of the project becomes clear. The word count of this type of abstract is generally more than descriptive abstract, but is usually less than 10% of the total length of the article (UNC-CH Writing Center, 2007).

Informative abstract with labeled sections are referred to as structured abstract (Hasselkus, 2001). Since its introduction into health science literatures in 1987, the use of structured abstract has gained popularity in the field (Ad Hoc Working Group for Critical Appraisal of the Medical Literature, 1987; Bayley & Eldredge, 2003). In the context of healthcare professionals, the use of this kind of abstract assists them in selecting clinically relevant and methodologically valid journal articles (National Library of Medicine, 2009).

It is observed that informative abstract is gaining popularity. This phenomenon is especially true in the nursing field. Although official statistics and research were not conducted, referring to the everyday experience of reading journals, use of informative or even structured abstract is frequently observed in clinical nursing research. Some journals, like *Nursing Research*, require authors to write structured abstracts for their articles.

## Structure and Components of Informative Abstract

An informative abstract is a complete story by itself. Regardless of the discipline of study and writing format, components of an informative abstract should encompass the following.

Background information of study gives brief description of the problems or issues that lead to the conduction of study. It would be imperative to address the gap of knowledge in this part. The purpose of study should be followed after addressing the knowledge gap, and research questions or hypothesis given in short statement should be included (Pierson, 2004).

Methodology part should follow. This part illustrates methods and instruments used in the study to resolve the problem or issue in simple words. In addition to the method, the setting, number of participants, selection criteria of participants, procedure and interventions should also be stated (Price, 2008). The reason for this is to reassure the reader that the study is properly conducted and is of good validity and reliability. The results that describe newly consolidated information would follow the methodology part. It provides data that is relevant to answer the research question (Cole & Koziol-McLain, 1997). If the study is a quantitative one, statistical analysis, for example, the mean score, statistical tests used should be reported. It is important to make sure that results reported in abstract are also reported in the body (Foote, 2006).

The conclusion or the implication part interprets the finding of study and states some useful implications derived from the study (Foote, 2006). It should be specific to the study and supportable to the findings of the study (Pierson, 2004). It should be avoided that the interpretations are more than what the results can support. Recommendations for further research or action can be given following the conclusion part. In short, informative abstract is not only a succinct collection of sentences, but a complete story with good structure and coherence.

# Abstract Writing in Nursing Journals

The writing requirement for the research paper to be published is usually indicated in the guidelines for authors. Different nursing journals come up with their own sets of writing guidelines. These guidelines may exhibit similarities, and yet there are some differences. Therefore, to get published in nursing journals, not only the content, but also the writing style of the abstract should be up to the requirements and criteria set by individual journals. In this context, guidelines for writing abstract in two different nursing journals, *Clinical Nursing Research* and *Nursing Research* (Nursing Research, 2009) are compared. By identifying the similarities and differences, this section illustrates the general requirements for getting published in nursing journals.

## The Structure of Abstract

Guideline of *Nursing Research* clearly indicates the structure of the abstract. Subsections of background, objectives, method, results and discussions should be included with the respective headings, i.e., use of structured abstract is preferred (Nursing Research, 2009). Requirements of individual subsections like number of sentences in a section, desired contents, are also listed in the guideline. For example, the background section has to summarize the literature review in one sentence and yet indicate the need for the study; objectives section has to state the hypothesis or main questions in the study in one sentence (*Nursing Research*, 2009).

Guideline of *Clinical Nursing Research* lists similar requirements and desires to have purpose, methodology, major results, and application included in the abstract (*Clinical Nursing Research*, 2009). Yet, it is less rigidly set as there is no indicated requirement for each subsection and there is no compulsory use of subheading for each subsection. Therefore, in general, abstract submitted for nursing journals should be well structured, regardless of whether the use of subheading is required.

Furthermore, guidelines of *Nursing Research* require author to include discussion section in the abstract (*Nursing Research*, 2009). According to the guidelines, the discussion part should be written based on the results found and has to include any implications or further studies (*Nursing Research*, 2009). On the other hand, *Clinical Nursing Research* requires only reporting of the results and any application from the study (*Clinical Nursing Research*, 2009). Just by going through the wording, apparently the requirements are different for the two journals. But if the author has to summarize the application in abstract, thorough understanding and in-depth interpretation of the results are required. Therefore, in this context, the content, no matter in the discussion part of *Nursing Research*, or the application part of *Clinical Nursing Research*, ought to be similar in terms of the requirement to interpret the results.

## Word Limit of Abstract

Apparently, there is no clear cut word limit of abstract for *Nursing Research*, but the abstract is required to be within one page with double-line spacing. In other words, the word count is estimated to be around 200, with the use of word processing software. Moreover, the number of sentences in each part is confined. For instance, background should be in one sentence, method should finish in three to four sentences.

Abstracts for *Clinical Nursing Research* should be even more concise. There is a strict word count of less than 150 words for abstracts in *Clinical Nursing Research* (*Clinical Nursing Research*, 2009). Within this limited number of words, the author is required to put down all the information designated. Though not having a guideline as strict as the previous journal, the author writing for *Clinical Nursing Research* should be able to manipulate the content well so as to achieve the best effects. Thus, in this sense, the abstract ought to be very succinct and yet indicate the most important sentences. One can say writing an abstract to be a challenge of language power.

## Inclusion of Keywords

Including keywords helps readers to search for the articles more easily. It is not a must in abstracts. In determining whether to include them or not, authors should refer to the guidelines of individual journals. *Clinical Nursing Research* indicated no requirement for inclusion of keywords. In contrast, the journal, *Nursing Research*, requires the author to put down two to three keywords specific to the study (*Nursing Research*, 2009). In addition, the words of choice are desired to be in a fashion indicated in the Medical Subject Headings (MeSH) guidelines.

MeSH is the vocabulary thesaurus controlled by the National Library of Medicine in the U.S. Its introduction is aimed at indexing article from 5,200 biomedical journals for the large well-known databases like the MEDLINE and PubMED (National Library of Medicine, 2008). The heading terms are arranged in a hierarchical order, which permits searching at various level of specificity (National Library of Medicine, 2008). Owing to the linkage of the journal with the databases, inclusion of such key words permits people to search the article through these databases easily.

## Other Considerations in Writing Abstracts

The abstract should be written in a manner that is friendly to those who are non-professional to the topic being investigated (Koopman, 1997). It cannot be assumed that the reader to be an expert on the topic conducted. Therefore, professional jargon or unnecessary abbreviations should be avoided in writing abstracts (Price, 2008). Abbreviations or acronyms in the abstract should be spelled out the first time they appear (Pierson, 2004). Generally, citations in the abstract section are not required. In both journals discussed, authors need not put down any references.

The content of the abstract should reflect the content of the article. International Committee of Medical Journal Editors (2009) discovered that the contents of many abstracts are different from that of the main article. Also, Vrijhoef and Steuten (2007) found that 18-68% of 264 abstracts from six major general medical journals were shown to contain data that were either inconsistent with or absent from the main article. Abstracts should not be exaggerating and, even worse, inaccurate. This gives no advantage to the article submitted and would actually mislead the readers.

# Implications for Nursing Authors

To get published in academic journals, including in the field of clinical nursing, crafting a good abstract is an essential. Although the abstract is often written after the main article is finished and relatively less time is spent on the writing of it, it is often the part frequently accessed by the readers.

The authors should pay attention to following key points summarized. Journals of nursing mainly accept informative or even structured abstracts, which provide more information when compared to descriptive abstracts. Informative abstracts should include concise sections of background, purpose of study, method, results and conclusion. In addition, some journals might set word limits or might require authors to match a few MeSH keywords with their articles. Besides, authors should be aware of the language used and the appropriateness of the use of abbreviations. A good abstract also means the ability to reflect the main article without exaggeration.

Good abstracts facilitate publication. There is no absolute guarantee of getting published in nursing journals even with a well-written abstract because worthiness of publication on nursing journals depends on the quality of the work.

# Conclusions

Well-written abstracts are essential for every single research article, regardless of the discipline or profession. Abstract writing in nursing research is also undeniably important. In addition to paying attention to the aforementioned factors, authors should refer closely to the guidelines set by the various journals.

In countries like the U.K. and the U.S., there are numerous academic and professional organizations of high academic status, like the American Psychology Association, International Committee of Medical Journal Editors, and so on. They establish internationally recognized writing guidelines. Besides, journals of high impact factors, like *Science* and *Nature*, all have definite guidelines and criteria set to authors who wish to publish their work.

Currently, Hong Kong lacks medical and nursing journals of high impact factor. Through using "Google," the popular search engine, attempts to access various local journals of medicine were made by using key word "Hong Kong Journal." It was found that only a few journals have set writing guidelines to authors. Having a well-written guideline for articles does not necessarily promote the impact factor of a journal. However, having a good control of the contents is a fundamental to a good quality journal. Therefore, regardless of the subjects or professions, local journals should set clear writing guidelines for the authors.

# Author's Background

Hung Fung was previously a biochemist and obtained his degree in biochemistry from The Chinese University of Hong Kong. He is now a candidate for the Master of Nursing pre-registration programme organized by the Hong Kong Polytechnic University.

# References

Ad Hoc Working Group for Critical Appraisal of the Medical Literature (1987). A proposal for more informative abstracts of clinical articles. *Ann. Intern. Med.* 106, 595 – 604.

Bayley, L. & Eldredge, J. (2003). The structured abstract: an essential tool for researchers. *Hypothesis.* 17 (1), 11 – 13.

Clinical Nursing Research (2009). Manuscript specifications for Clinical Nursing Research. Retrieved on 12th November, 2009 from http://www.sagepub.com/journalsProdManSub.nav?prodId=Journal200890.

Cole, F. L. & Koziol-McLain, J. (1997). Writing a research abstract. *Journal of Emergency Nursing.* 23(5), 487 – 490.

Cole, J. (2008). Mastering the Abstract Writing Process. Retrieved on 12th November, 2009 from http://www.societyforscience.org/Document.Doc?id=27.

Colorado State University (2009). Writing Abstracts: Types of Abstracts— Descriptive Abstract. Retrieved on 11th November, 2009 from http://writing.colostate.edu/guides/documents/abstract/list5.cfm.

Costa-Pierce, B. (1997). Writing a Smashing Abstract Takes Practice! Retrieved on 12th November, 2009 from http://darwin.bio.uci.edu/~sustain/Abstract.html.

Fisher, W. E. (2005). Abstract Writing. *Journal of Surgical Research.* 128, 162 – 164.

Foote, M. (2006). Some Concrete Ideas about Manuscript Abstracts. *Chest.* 129(5), 1375 – 1377.

Hasselkus, B. R. (2001). Writing the Abstract: The Most Important Part of the Manuscript? *The American Journal of Occupational Therapy.* 55(2), 127 - 128.

International Committee of Medical Journal Editors (2009). Uniform Requirements for Manuscripts Submitted to Biomedical Journals: Manuscript Preparation and Submission: Preparing a Manuscript for Submission to a Biomedical Journal. Retrieved on 11th November, 2009 from http://www.icmje.org/manuscript_1prepare.html.

International Council of Nurses (2009). Nursing Research. Geneva: ICN.

Killborn, J. (1998). Writing Abstracts. Retrieved on 10th November, 2009 from http://leo.stcloudstate.edu/bizwrite/abstracts.html.

Koopman, P. (1997). How to Write an Abstract. Retrieved on 11th November, 2009 from http://www.ece.cmu.edu/~koopman/essays/abstract.html.

National Library of Medicine (2008). Medical Subject Heading Factsheet. Retrieved on 11th November, 2009 from http://www.nlm.nih.gov/pubs/factsheets/mesh.html.

National Library of Medicine (2009). Structured Abstracts: What are structured abstracts? Retrieved online on 11th November, 2009 from http://www.nlm.nih.gov/bsd/policy/structured_abstracts.html.

Nursing Research (2009). Information for Authors. Retrieved on 12th November, 2009 from http://edmgr.ovid.com/nres/accounts/ifauth.htm.

Pierson, D. J. (2004). How to Write an Abstract That Will Be Accepted for Presentation at a National Meeting. *Respiratory Care*, 49(10), 1206 – 1210.

Price, C. (2008). Writing an Abstract. Retrieved on 11th November, 2009 from http://www.aspan.org/Portals/6/docs/Research/Writing_an_Abstract. pdf.

UNC-CH Writing Center (2007). Retrieved on 10th November, 2009 from http://www.unc.edu/depts/wcweb/handouts/abstracts.html.

University of California Berkeley (1997). How to write an abstract. Retrieved on 12th November, 2009 from http://research.berkeley.edu/ucday/ abstract.html.

Vrijhoef, H. J. M. & Steuten, L. M. G. (2007). How to write an abstract. *European Diabetes Nursing.* 4(3), 124 - 127.

In: Clinical Research Issues in Nursing          ISBN: 978-1-61668-937-7
Editor: Z. C. Y. Chan, pp.13-22          © 2010 Nova Science Publishers, Inc.

*Chapter II*

# The Art of Abstract Writing for Nursing Research

*Mary W. S. Mok and*
*Zenobia C. Y. Chan*
The Hong Kong Polytechnic University, China

## Abstract

A growing expectation on nurses to utilize research findings for daily practice leads to an increased demand for nurses to sharpen their research skills. Abstract writing is a component of research skills and is one of the important steps. A well-written abstract is vital in communicating the research findings to others, which is a key objective for doing research. This paper explains the importance of the abstract, its structure and anatomy, and ways to contribute to a quality abstract. Requirements of two nursing journals' abstract methods are used to discuss the different structures and approaches to abstract writing. The objective for this chapter is not only to discuss the technical aspect of abstract writing, but also the art of abstract writing. It delivers a clear message to researchers about the importance of developing passionate skills in the art of abstract writing, as well as being knowledgeable regarding the structure and requirements of the abstract.

# Introduction

Nursing is a profession that requires continuous growth in practice and knowledge. Each nurse has the role and responsibility to participate in research activities ranging from reading research articles, applying the research findings into daily practice and actively participating in research studies. Involvement in research is essential in the nursing profession. Nursing research provides opportunities for continuous professional growth and development. It also contributes to the improvement in the quality of nursing care, thus promoting patients' optimal outcomes (Mirr Jansen & Zwygart-Stauffacher, 2006). The goal for research is to formulate conclusions and to communicate the findings to others. Therefore, the potential readers can access and learn the new knowledge through the published research articles. Although communicating the findings of research study is the last step in research process, it is an important step in achieving the goal of the study (LoBiondo-Wood & Haber, 1998; Polit, Beck, & Hungler, 2001). A research abstract plays an important role in this step to capture the interest of the potential readers in that it is the first section and can be the only section the readers read. It should be well organized, structured, and written to capture the interest of potential readers. Research abstracts may be difficult to write, especially for the novice researchers; however, they should put forth an effort to follow the path for a well-written research abstract.

A well-written research abstract requires good abstract writing skills. Abstract writing is similar to the art and science of the nursing practice. Knowledge of the importance, requirements, and components of a research abstract underlie the science of abstract writing. Researchers are required to have sufficient knowledge on the science of abstract writing as a foundation to prepare a well-written abstract. The art of abstract writing is the mental and cognitive task for abstracting and abstract writing. A well-written abstract requires the author's passion, time and effort in abstract writing.

In Day's preface (1979), he advised the authors of scientific papers:

> There are four things that make this world go round: love, energy, materials, and information. We see about us a critical shortage of the first commodity, a near-critical shortage of the second, increasing shortage of the third, but an absolute glut of the fourth (p iii).

Nurse researchers need to develop skills and devote time into producing a clear, precise and refined abstract; so that it can deliver the greatest possible amount of information within the specified length of an abstract (Cremmins, 1982; Fisher, 2005). Both the art and science of abstract writing are essential for a quality, well-written and successful research abstract.

This chapter will explain the purpose of a research abstract and the time for writing it. The types, structures and components of an abstract and its characteristics will be discussed as well as illustrated by the comparison of two nursing research journals' requirements for abstract writing. In addition to the fundamental knowledge in writing an abstract, reading and cognitive skills for abstracting and abstract writing skills will also be discussed in this chapter.

# Purpose of a Research Abstract

A research abstract is a concise and comprehensive summary, being placed at the beginning of an article, which communicates the essential ideas of the project (Cole & Koziol-McLain, 1997; Fink & Oman 2003; Fisher, 2005). It summarizes the article's contents and compiles its key points. The abstract is as important as the body of the article, and it serves multiple functions in communicating the research study. It is a determining factor in promoting the article for publication. The quality of an abstract gives a first impression to the experienced editors in determining the acceptance of the article for publication in their journals (Brazier, 1997; Fisher, 2005). Further, the abstract of a published article may appear in a search database such as CINAHL or MEDLINE. It is an important channel for the potential readers to access the articles in the information-retrieval system (Brown, 1989). The information-retrieval system is the main mechanism of the articles being posted and used by the potential readers (Fisher, 2005). There is a very small number of readers who will read the whole article; the majority will read the abstract first (Brazier, 1997). The abstract allows the readers to assess the article and identify its content quickly and accurately to determine its relevance to their interests. The readers' decisions in making their efforts to read the entire article will largely be based on the quality of the abstract. (Brazier 1997; Evans, 1994; Fisher 2005). Therefore, a well-written abstract is vital in attracting the potential readers to consult the full article.

# When to Write the Abstract

The timing for abstract writing is one of the crucial elements in producing a well-written abstract. Although the anatomy of a research article is that the abstract is placed at the beginning of it, there are diverse practices or preferences in the time to write an abstract. An abstract is the concise summary of the full article (Day, 1979). It should be written when the study findings are completely understood and after the completion of the article in order to promote and enhance the accuracy of the abstract. This approach can ensure a full reflection of the article in the abstract (Brazier, 1997; Hasselkus, 2001). Whether the authors write the abstract before or after the completion of an article, they should be knowledgeable on the types, structures, and components of an abstract.

# Types of Abstracts

Abstracts often are classified by their content, purpose and structure (Cremmins, 1982). Indicative and informative are the two main types of abstracts. An indicative or descriptive abstract can indicate the subjects being dealt with in a paper similar to a table of contents. However, it contains information only on the purpose, scope, or methodology of a research study that just simply describes what the article contains. Therefore, it can seldom be used as a representation for the full research article because of its descriptive nature. An informative abstract is also designed to condense the paper and be a reflection of the full article. In addition to the information included in indicative abstracts, informative abstracts also contain the research results, conclusions, or recommendations (Cremmins, 1982; Day, 1998; Hasselkus, 2001; Tornquist, 1986). The aim of a nursing research study and its article is to communicate the new finding or knowledge to readers as well as to contribute to the body of nursing knowledge. An informative abstract is preferred for a research article, as it is not only contains information on the research study but also on what the study contributes. The results, conclusions, and recommendations included in the informative abstract are necessary in communicating the new findings to the readers.

# Structure of an Abstract

An informative abstract is chosen and used to summarize a research article because of its substantive nature. However, different research journals may have their own requirements on the structure of abstract. The difference in their requirements will be illustrated by a comparison of two nursing research journals, *Clinical Nursing Research* and *American Journal of Critical Care*, in this section. The golden rule for an article being accepted for publication is to follow the journals' requirements (Brazier, 1997; Evans, 1994). It is the author's responsibility to ensure the format of his abstract and other components of an article follow the requirements thoroughly. Structured abstracts require authors to write their abstracts to subsections for the key aspects of purpose, methods, and results in a standardized format (Brazier, 1997; Quinn & Rush, 2009). Informal or unstructured abstracts contain the same information as structured abstracts, but they are just organized in one long narrative paragraph (Quinn & Rush, 2009). *Clinical Nursing Research* has the guidelines for the authors to prepare an informal abstract in a single paragraph for the summary of the article including its purpose, methodology, major results and application, if appropriate. The format requirement of an abstract for the *American Journal of Critical Care* is a structured abstract with background, objective, methods, results, and conclusions as the subheadings. The requirements of abstract structure for the two nursing research journals serve the same purpose of abstract writing. Both structure requirements can condense and concentrate the essential information in an article. Therefore, authors should prepare the abstract in the same way for an informal abstract cognitively; even headings are not required. This practice can ensure that there no important elements of the article are omitted. The authors also need to have a structure in mind while writing the informal abstract. This can help them to identify and summarize the key features of their work (Brazier, 1997). As a novice nurse researcher, I find it is easier to read and retrieve the important details of the article and to assess the applicability of the study from a structured abstract.

# Components of an Abstract

The authors should stay focused on the essential components for research abstract whether they need to prepare a structured or informal abstract. The typical components are title, introduction and background, purpose and objectives, methodology, results, and conclusion (Boswell, Cannon & Holden-Hucton, 2004; Brazier, 1997; Cole & Koziol-McLain, 1997; Fink & Oman, 2003; Lindquist, 1993; Shaughnessy, 2009). The abstract title should reflect the nature of the research study and be coherent to the content of the abstract to promote others' interest in reading the abstract. Begin the abstract with a background statement about the nature of the research problem and to provide the rationale for the study. The importance of the study and theoretical framework should also be included, as framework provides structure and guidance for understanding the complexity of the research problems. The body of the abstract should be a brief and clear statement on the objective of the study, including the study purpose, specific aims, research questions, or hypothesis (Boswell, Cannon, & Holden-Hucton, 2004; Fink & Oman 2003). The setting, study population, sample selection, and research design should also be identified and included. The result is likely to be the longest section in the abstract that provides the observations being made from the research study (Brazier, 1997). Interpretation of the results should only take place in the abstract conclusion section. The abstract should conclude with clinical implications based on the findings and data from the study (Cole & Koziol-McLain 1997; Fink & Oman 2003). Many literatures support that an abstract title should be one of the components of abstract. However, both nursing research journals, *Clinical Nursing Research* and *American Journal of Critical Care*, do not include an abstract title as their requirement for abstract formulation. These two journals require authors to send their articles with abstracts for peer review. Therefore, a title page for the article is required instead of an abstract title, and they have specifications for the title of an article as well.

# Characteristics of a Good Research Abstract

A well-written abstract serves as a guide to the full article that provides the reader with an initial understanding of the published research article. A well-written abstract should be accurate, self-contained, concise and specific, non-evaluative, coherent and readable. Abstracts are expected to be accurate, as readers depend on its content to determine whether proceed to read the entire article. The content and purpose of the article should be precisely and fully reflected in the abstract. Data and findings obtained should be mentioned consistently between the abstract and the body of the article. Only the information from the article should be included in the abstract to guarantee its accuracy (Boswell, Cannon, & Holden-Hucton, 2004; Brown, 1989; Hasselkus, 2001). Being self-contained is also a characteristic of a well-written abstract. All the abbreviations, acronyms, and unique terms used in the abstract need to be well defined. Quotations are not acceptable. Key words should also be included in the abstract for indexing purposes (Boswell, Cannon, & Holden-Hucton, 2004; Brown, 1989). Embedding key concepts, words, and phrases in the abstract will ensure the article is properly indexed. Careful choosing on the wording for the abstract is necessary. The authors should consider the point of view of the readers who try to retrieve information from the search databases. It increases the chance for the readers to find the article from the database by using similar concepts and terms that appear in the abstract (Brazier, 1997).

Conciseness and specificity is also an expectation for all abstract submissions. All sentences should be as informative and brief as possible to include only the most important findings and data. Word count should within the limit requirement of the journals (Brown, 1989). A submission of a 6,200-word research article to *Clinical Nursing Research* requires a maximum of a 150-word informal abstract. In comparison, *American Journal of Critical Care* requires a structured abstract of no more than 250 words for a research article with 1,500 to 4,000 words. *Clinical Nursing Research* requires a more concise abstract than *American Journal of Critical Care*. An abstract should be non-evaluative. It should only report, but not evaluate, the findings and data obtained in the research study. The final, but not the least, characteristic of a well-written abstract is that it is coherent and readable. A clear and vigorous writing style is best for message delivery and to capture the interest of readers (Boswell, Cannon, & Holden-Hucton, 2004; Brown, 1989). The challenge in writing a quality abstract is that it should be comprehensive and brief at the same time. A well-conceived and executed research study can fail in publication if its abstract is not well focused or is poorly written. Therefore, nurse researchers should not only equip themselves with research skills, but also strengthen their abstract writing skills.

# Implications for Nursing Research

A well-written abstract cannot be written without good abstract writing skills. The abstract is probably one of the most difficult sections to write. It is a possible obstacle for nurse researchers to complete their research process as well as to communicate their findings to the public through publication. Therefore, nurse researchers should strengthen their skills in abstract writing. The art aspect of abstract writing, including reading, analytical thinking and technical writing skills, can be developed through experience and practice. Critical reading skills are required to determine the characteristics and important features of content to be abstracted as well as to identify relevant information from the article. A strong analytical thinking skill is required to extract information cognitively before formulating and writing the abstract. Well-developed English technical writing skills are essential to a well-written abstract (Cremmins, 1982; Widerquist, 2000). It can use words and their meanings to form the fundamental component of knowledge as well as to deliver message to readers effectively. Besides having adequate knowledge and skills in abstract writing, the researchers should also spend energy and put effort into writing (Day, 1979). The more energy the researcher spends in abstract writing, the less energy required from the reader to obtain the relevant information from the abstract. Day (1979) also advises that they need to love the English language and need to engage in reading and writing more literature that is English. It is important for nurse researchers to keep reading and to enjoy the reading of others' research writing. This is not only to develop their own reading skills, experience in abstracting and writing abstract, but also to develop their habit in loving the English language and research studies.

# Conclusion

The current trend in nursing professional is to apply evidence-based practice in daily practice. There are more nurses who undertake research projects to improve the performance in clinical settings in order to achieve a better clinical practice, and subsequently, with a better patient outcome. This move provides us the opportunity and responsibility to share our findings with others (Shaughnessy, 2009). The result of a research study always inspires new ideas and leads to new research questions (Portney & Watkins, 2009). A well-written abstract is invaluable to the research author, in that it aids the publication process as well as encourages others to read their works. As a result, the new knowledge from the study can add to the knowledge pool. Understanding the importance, requirements, and art of abstract writing are the essential components of a well-written abstract. The abstract deserves the same amount of energy and effort that is devoted to the body of the article. It may be the last section to be written, but it should not be the least priority in research writing (Hasselkus, 2001). The researchers should not neglect the importance and power of a well-written abstract, as it can help them to achieve their research goals in publishing their articles and expanding the knowledge in nursing profession.

## Author's Background

Mary Mok Wing Sze is a Master Nursing student studying in the Hong Kong Polytechnic University. (Email: mokwingsze@gmail.com).

## References

American Association of Critical-Care Nurses. (2009). *Author Guidelines for American Journal of Critical Care.* Retrieved Nov 20, 2009, from American Journal of Critical Care: http://ajcc.aacnjournals.org/misc/AJCCAuthGuide.pdf.

Boswell, C., Cannon, S., & Holden-Hucton, P. (2004). Developing Abstracts for Workshops and Conferences: Improve Your Chance of Acceptance. *Nursing Education Perspectives, 25(1)*, 10-11.

Brazier, H. (1997). Writing a research abstract: structure, style and content. *Nursing Standard, 11(48)*, 34-36.

Brown, J. M. (1989). Driven to Abstraction: Writing an Abstract for Presentation or Publication. *Journal of Intravenous Nursing, 12(5)*, 326-328.

Cole, F., & Koziol-McLain, J. (1997). Writing a research abstract. *Journal of Emergency Nursing, 23(5)*, 487-490.

Cremmins, E. T. (1982). *The Art of Abstracting.* Philadelphia: ISI Press.

Day, R. A. (1979). *How to Write & Publish a Scientific Paper.* Philadelphia: ISI Press.

Evans, J. C. (1994). The Art of Writing Successful Research Abstracts. *Neonatal Network, 13(5)*, 49-52.

Fink, R. M., & Oman, K. S. (2003). *Writing a Research Abstract.* Philadelphia: Hanley & Belfus, Inc.

Fisher, W. E. (2005). Astract Writing. *Journal of Surgical Research, 128(2)*, 162-164.

Hasselkus, B. R. (2001). Writing the Abstract: The Most Important Part of the Manuscript. *The American Journal of Occupational Therapy, 55(2)*, 127-128.

Lindquist, R. A. (1993). Strategies for Writing A Competitive Research Abstract. *Dimensions of Critical Care Nursing, 12(1)*, 46-53.

LoBiondo-Wood, G., & Haber, J. (1998). *Nursing Research. Methods, Critical Appraisal, and Utilization. (4th ed.).* St. Louis: Mosby.

Mirr Jansen, M. P., & Zwygart-Stauffacher, M. (2006). *Advanced Practice Nursing. Core Concepts for Professional Role Development. (3rd ed.).* New York: Springer Publishing Company.

Polit, D. F., Beck, C. T., & Hungler, B. P. (2001). *Essential of Nursing Research. Methods, Appraisal, and Utilization. (5th ed.).* Philadelphia: Lippincott Williams & Wilkins.

Portney, L. G., & Watkins, M. P. (2009). *Foundations of clinical research: application to practice, (3rd ed.).* New Jersey: Pearson Education, Inc.

Quinn, C. T., & Rush, J. A. (2009). Writing and Publishing Your Research Findings. *Journal of Investigative Medicine, 57(5)*, 634-639.

SAGE Publication. (2009). *Manuscript Sepcifications for Clinical Nursing Research.* Retrieved Dec 2, 2009, from SAGE Publication: http://www.sagepub.com/journalsProdManSub.nav?prodId=Journal200890

Shaughnessy, M. (2009). Abstracts That Score! *Geriatric Nursing, 30(2)*, 141-142.

Tornquist, E. M. (1986). *From Proposal to Publication. An Informal Guide to Writing about Nursing Research.* California: Addison-Wesley Publishing Company.

Widerquist, J. G. (2000). Abstract Writing. *Hospital Material Management Quarterly, 122(2)*, 58-63.

In: Clinical Research Issues in Nursing  ISBN: 978-1-61668-937-7
Editor: Z. C. Y. Chan, pp.23-32  © 2010 Nova Science Publishers, Inc.

*Chapter III*

# Abstract Writing in Nursing Research

## *H. M. Shek and*
## *Zenobia C.Y. Chan*
The Hong Kong Polytechnic University, China

## Abstract

An abstract is a comprehensive description of a research study. Since an abstract has a maximum word limit, it can be difficult for authors to outline the most significant aspects of the work. Therefore, despite clinical research technique, abstract writing skills are also important for the nurse researcher. The content and presentation of a research abstract can greatly influence the acceptance of a research article for publication. However, there are only a few nursing research articles focusing on abstract writing and none in Hong Kong. It seems that nurses in Hong Kong can be more active in clinical research when compared to the Western countries. The purpose of writing this chapter is to attract the interest of nurses, particularly nurses in Hong Kong, in abstract writing and consequently stimulates their motivation in performing clinical research.

# Introduction

An abstract appears at the beginning of an article. It is a concise and a condense description of a research study. An abstract is a medium to disseminate the research and conveys the significant ideas to readers in order to decide if the article is of interest of them (Parahoo, 1997). Sometimes, there is a misconception between an abstract and an introduction since both of them present the research problem and objectives as well as briefly reviewing methodology, main findings and conclusions. An introduction aims to introduce the research area by presenting its context, the research problem, and how it will be examined. In contrast, an abstract tends to summarize the whole research. Juhi and Norman (1989) stated that an abstract is to declare the purpose of the research, the method of study employed, and other important aspects of the work, including the findings and conclusions (p.189). In addition, an abstract follows the criteria of a specific journal (Brazier, 1997; Heppner & Heppner, 2004; Waston, 2006). An abstract should be readable and precisely highlight the content of the research article. Therefore, a well-constructed abstract requires comprehensive planning. Planning is similar to other work of art that is achieved in stages (Evans, 1994). In this essay, it will first explore the importance and art of an abstract writing. Then it will delineate the key elements involved in a research abstract. In addition, two nursing journals' requirements for abstract will be compared and described. Furthermore, it will also discuss the implications and suggestions of abstract writing to nursing in Hong Kong.

This chapter consists of six main parts: a) Key elements of a research abstract; b) Significance of a research abstract; c) Art of abstract writing; d) Structured and unstructured abstract; e) Implications for nursing research; and f) Conclusion.

# Key Elements of a Research Abstract

Each nursing organization has its particular criteria for abstract writing. In general, abstracts vary in length from 50 to 250 words, and references are excluded in an abstract. It also varies among journal organizations. The major components of a research abstract include problem or purpose, methodology, results, and conclusions or clinical implications.

## Title

The title introduces the topic area of the research project. In addition, it is an advertising instrument of a study. An interesting title can attract attention of reviewers who eventually continue to read the abstract and then the whole article. The title can be a question or a statement. However, any statement developed in the title must be supported by data within the article (Brazier, 1997; Cole & Koziol-McLain, 1997).

## Problem or Purpose

Problem or purpose can be a statement, a form of hypotheses, or a question that starts the text of an abstract. Indeed, it is the most important portion in an abstract since it provides a clear insight to readers in relation to the importance of the research problems, the rationales for the investigation, and the benefits of the project. Also, it can capture the reviewers' interest and eventually entices them to continue reading (Evans, 1994; Haller, 1988; Murdaugh, 1988).

## Methodology

Methodology is the description of the research design, for example an ethnography study or a post-test only control group design. Moreover, the selection of subjects, whether it is a random or a consecutive sampling, and the size of the study population should also be delineated. The sample characteristics such as age and gender are included in this section as well. Furthermore, the reliability and validity of research instruments used in data collection should be described in order to adjust the rigor of the research (Evans, 1994; Haller, 1988; Murdaugh, 1988).

## Results

Results are probably the longest section in a research abstract. It summarizes the key findings of both qualitative and quantitative key research studies. Significantly, the results should be consistent with the purpose of the abstract. However, interpretation of the results appears in the conclusion part (Cole & Koziol-McLain, 1997; Walker, 1986).

## Conclusions or Clinical Implications

A conclusion briefly describes the generalization of the findings, suggestions for future research, implications for nursing practice and establishment of theoretical framework (Cole & Koziol-McLain, 1997; Lindquist, 1993; Walker, 1986). The chief idea is often presented in the last sentence. It provides the answer to the question or purposes declared in the first part of the abstract. Nevertheless, the findings should relate to the problem and purpose of the study. In addition, the restatement of the findings should be prevented. On the other hand, any limitations that may influence the results of the project should be stated as well (Brazier, 1997).

Based on the above key elements, they provide a systematic description of a research study. For example, in methodology, it enables readers to recognize information such as study design, sample size, and method of selection. However, it is suggested to add detail relating to literature review in this section, for example, the databases and key words that have been used in the process of literature review.

# Significance of a Research Abstract

A research abstract is necessitated in almost all professional journals. An abstract is the first impression of a research article. It is also an advertisement to promote the research study to the editor, reviewers and potential readership to select the research project. An abstract is the initial part of the article that a reviewer will read (Waston, 2006). It is likely that a majority of readers will read the abstract instead of the whole article. An attractive abstract can capture the interest of the readers and help them decide whether to continue to read the entire paper. On the other hand, a research abstract is a valuable tool for those who are planning to conduct a research to identify the knowledge gap or the missing gap of their thesis and argument (Fuller, 1983; Haigh, 2006). It helps to save the reading time since the readers can know the research problem and its findings without reading the whole research paper. Moreover, selection of research articles for publication can be based on the content of an abstract. It allows the review committees to judge the quality and relevance of a research study. Nurse reviewers often rate the abstract according to some predetermined guidelines. Those highly rated abstracts will then be further considered as a publishable article (Cole & Koziol-McLain, 1997; Juhi & Norman, 1989; Stromborg, 1981). Furthermore, with the advancement of technology, the electronic search engines such as CINAHL, British Nursing Index, and Medline are commonly used to search for research articles. In the process of article research, there are hundreds of articles displayed for the search result. By reviewing the abstract of the articles, it enables the readers to recognize the key ideas of the research study and helps to identify the correct topics and articles for the users (Brazier, 1997; Haber & LoBiondo-Wood, 1994; Walker, 1986).

# Art of Abstract Writing

As mentioned before, there is a length restriction for a research abstract. As a result, a comprehensive planning is essential in order to create an abstract in a concise and accurate manner. Planning is an art of abstract writing. A successful planning of abstract writing consists of several stages. They are planning the abstract, draft, preliminary review, peer review, editing, and packing and will be discussed in the following (Evans, 1994).

## Planning

Planning is the outline formation of a research abstract. It concentrates in identification of necessary and unique contents involved in an abstract writing. An innovative abstract is highly probable to be accepted by a professional organization. Indeed, it might be easier to develop the outline by following the specific instructions from a professional organization. The instructions act as a backbone of an abstract. Most importantly, it assists the author to arrange the flow of abstract smoothly and to ascertain all requirements have been accomplished. The evaluation of a research abstract sometimes will be assessed on its synchronization with specific criteria from a professional organization, which may result in the abstract not being sent to the peer reviews or failure to grade the article (Lindquist, 1993; Walker, 1986).

## Draft

Draft is the connection of all items being established in the outline. In this stage, the major issues are determined and clarified. A well-developed abstract contributes to a well-presented paper (Brazier, 1997). In some circumstances, the length of an abstract may exceed the word limit. However, it is not the instant concern unless they are as precise as possible. The deduction of the words of a research abstract can be done in preliminary and peer revisions and editing (Murdaugh, 1988; Walker, 1986).

## Preliminary Review

Preliminary review is a content review. It aims to ascertain all required subject and major aspects are included in the research abstract. In addition, it determines whether the content flows glidingly from beginning to end, and the purpose is linked to the conclusions. In order to create an effective preliminary review, it is proposed to incubate the draft alone for at least three days as this provides time for reflection (Evans, 1994).

## Peer Review

Peer review is followed by preliminary review. The purpose of peer review is to measure how well a research study matches the idea and therefore to avoid the presentation of poor research. It is suggested that the draft can be evaluated by individuals who are familiar with the research study or those who are not. It is because each individual may have different connotations of the same word. More comments can positively improve the quality of research abstract (Murdaugh, 1988). Sometimes, it may be difficult to evaluate a research abstract with limited details. As a result, the selection of abstract reviewers should be based on their knowledge and their ability to give constructive feedback. The reviewers can be journal editors or the acknowledged experts in the profession. Once all the reviewers' comments have been returned, the author can highlight the comments that are significant, omit unnecessary items, decrease the length of an abstract within the limits, and refine the abstract correspondingly (Evans, 1994).

## Editing

Editing is comprised of spelling, typing, format accuracy, and inclusion of all contents according to the guidelines of a specific journal. In this circumstance, it is necessary to ensure all reported numbers and statistics are accurate. Furthermore, a proofreader can be selected to perform a double check on all details (Walker, 1986).

## Packaging

Packaging refers to the professional appearance of a research abstract. An abstract with an attractive and professional appearance provides a favorable impression for the reviewer. An abstract with spelling errors and sloppy text alignment or a poor quality of print may give reviewers a sense of carelessness, and they are likely to reject the article. Hence, it is important to have the final check of an abstract based on the journal instructions before submission (Lindquist, 1993).

# Structured and Unstructured Abstract

A research abstract can be structured or unstructured. A structured abstract refers to the components of the research study that are presented as headings in the abstract (Cole & Koziol-McLain, 1997). It is valuable to adopt a standardized format so that the author can easily and clearly communicate the main details of the research. In addition, it is easier for the reviewer to identify the major features of the research project (Hirai, Naito, Nakayama & Yamazaki, 2005; James, 2004). In contrast, there will be no subheadings in unstructured abstract. Perhaps, without a systemic approach it may cause an inaccurate abstract and fail to report the important content of the study. Accordingly, it is likely that an informal abstract is less informative than a structured abstract (Haller, 1992; Midwifery, 1994). The requirements of abstract writing of two nursing journals: *The Australian Journal of Advanced Nursing* and the *Journal Geronotological Nursing* will be discussed as follows.

*The Australian Journal of Advanced Nursing* requires a structured abstract to be presented under a series of headings. Clear guidelines are provided for each subheading. They guide the authors, in particular those who have the research idea but are unsure how to start wring up an abstract. A structured abstract provides a clear picture about the aspects that should be described in each subsection. Accordingly, any inappropriate data must be avoided and make the abstract as informative as possible. Besides, a structured abstract makes it easier for the reviewers' committee to choose the most suitable studies for publication.

In the *Journal of Gerontological Nursing*, the abstract only requires the author to present the findings and conclusions. In this circumstance, none of the research background details are stated. It is significant to realize the objective of the study and the design of the study. Moreover, it is also important to perceive the method of participant selection in order to adjust if they fit the investigation. As a result, it may be difficult to determine the validity and reliability of the research findings without a concrete description.

# Implications for Nursing Research

In recent years, evidence-based practice has become a popular issue in nursing practice. In other words, it is vital that the nursing practice is based on scientific evidence. Hong Kong will be an example for discussion. To further facilitate the development of nursing practice and enrich the body of nursing knowledge in Hong Kong, it is necessary to conduct research. An interesting and clear abstract may be able to stimulate the interests of nurses in Hong Kong towards research. It is the responsibilities of nurses to expand their knowledge base and keep evaluating the most updated information regarding health care issues. This helps to provide a high quality of care and minimize the incidence of medical errors. All these can be achieved by reviewing research articles or performing research. Moreover, once nurses develop skills in abstract writing, they may become more confident in writing a research article. Hence, it increases their motivations to conduct research. As more nurses conduct research and publish their works, the research basis of nursing in Hong Kong will become stronger. Perhaps, Hong Kong can develop a nursing journal organization to encourage and assist nurses in performing clinical research. The organization can be under universities, hospital authority, or private nursing agencies. In addition, the organization can invite experienced researchers, nurse specialists and involve young scholars to formulate some protocols in writing English and Chinese journal articles. Besides, the organization can organize several workshops to train and encourage nurses to conduct clinical research. It is also anticipated that Hong

Kong can establish a local abstract writing requirements, in both English and Chinese abstracts.

# Conclusion

An abstract summarizes the major contents of research. It serves to introduce reviewers to the chief points of a study. Moreover, it is also an advertisement tool to promote the research. A well-presented abstract should be readable, concise, accurate, and able to capture the interest of readers. On the other hand, it should be consistent with the guidelines of a nursing journal organization. To be successful in abstract writing, a careful planning is essential. Furthermore, it is believed that a structured abstract is more informative than an unstructured abstract. A structured abstract assists authors to identify the most significant information of the study. It is expected that Hong Kong can develop its own nursing journal organization and abstract writing guidelines. It is no doubt that the acceptance of a research article for publication always requires an effective abstract writing skill.

# Author's Background

Shek Hei Man is a year two student of Master of Nursing in the Hong Kong Polytechnic University. (Email: spongefinger1983@yahoo.com.hk)

# References

Brazier, H. (1997). Writing a research abstract structure: Structure, style and content. *Nursing Standard, 11* (48), 34-36.

Cole, F.L. & Koziol-McLain, J. (1997). The research column: Writing a research abstract. *Journal of Emergency Nursing, 23* (5), 487-490.

Evans, J.C. (1994). The art of writing a successful research abstracts. *Neonatal Network, 13* (5), 49-52.

Fuller, E.O. (1983) Preparing an abstract of a nursing study. *Nursing Research, 32* (5), 316-317.

Haber, J. & Lobiondo-Wood, G. (1994). *Nursing research: Methods, critical appraisal, and utilization (3$^{rd}$ ed)*. Missouri: Mosby.

Haigh, C.A. (2006). The art of the abstract. *Nurse Education Today, 26* (5), 355-357.

Haller, K.B. (1988). Writing effective research abstracts. *The American Journal of Maternal Child Nursing, 13* (1), 74.

Haller, K.B. (1992). Changing our style: Adopting a familiar publication style and introducing informative abstracts. *Journal of Obstetric, Gynecologic & Neonatal Nursing, 21* (1), 11.

Hartley, J. (2004). Current findings from research on structured abstracts. *Journal of the Medical Library Association, 92* (3), 368-371.

Happner, M.J. & Heppner, P.P. (2004). *Writing and publishing your thesis, dissertation & research: A guide for students in the helping professions.* Belmont: Thomson Learning, Inc.

Hirai, N.; Naito, M.; Nakayama T. & Yamazaki S. (2005). Adoption of structured abstracts by general medical journals and format for a structured abstract. *Journal of the Medical Library Association, 93* (2), 237-242.

Journal of Gerontological Nursing (2009). *Information for contributors.* Retrieved November 31, 2009 from http://www.jognonline.com/about.asp

Juhi, N. & Norman, V.L. (1989). Writing an effective abstract. *Applied Nursing research, 2* (4), 189-193.

Lindquist, R.A. (1993). Strategies for writing a competitive research abstract. *Dimensions of Critical Care Nursing, 12* (1), 46-53.

Midwifery. (1994). A change in the presentation of abstracts. *Midwifery, 10,* 58.

Murdaugh, C.M. (1988). Writing a research abstract. *Progress in Cardiovascular Nursing, 3,* 98-100.

Parahoo, K. (1997). *Nursing research: Principles, process and issues.* Hampshire: Macmillan Press, Ltd.

Stromborg, M. & Wegmann, J. (1981). The fine art of writing a research abstract. *Oncology Nursing Forum, 8* (4), 67-71.

The Australian Journal of Advanced Nursing. (2009). *Author guidelines.* Retrieved November 31, 2009 from http://www.ajan.com.au/ajan_guidelines. html.

Walker, S.N. (1986). Less is more: Writing an abstract of nursing research. *CHART, 83,* 8-9.

Waston, R. (2009). *Writing an abstract.* Retrieved November 31, 2009 from http://www.nurseauthoreditor.com/article.asp?id=60.

In: Clinical Research Issues in Nursing
Editor: Z. C. Y. Chan, pp.33-41

ISBN: 978-1-61668-937-7
© 2010 Nova Science Publishers, Inc.

*Chapter IV*

# Literature Review in Nursing Research: The Importance and the Practical Guidelines

## S. K. Lai and Zenobia C.Y. Chan

The Hong Kong Polytechnic University, China

## Abstract

In this chapter, the importance of nursing literature review and the method to write it systematically in a practical way is discussed. This chapter integrates the ideas of how literature review should be conducted and produced from a number of nursing research books. It aims at producing a clear and simple framework for researchers who start to write nursing literature review. Also, the guidelines for nursing literature review are provided in a comprehensive and easy to understand manner in this chapter. Evidence-based practice is essential to improve quality of existing nursing care. Literature review is vital to the profession's development as it gives evidence to researches that help to perfect nursing care. This chapter is written in hope of promoting the development of the nursing profession.

# Introduction

Literature review in nursing research has two important natures. Firstly, it is part of the text of a research paper. It is a large part of an academic research paper, which usually precedes the methodology, result and discussion parts. In a research paper, its main role is to review the current knowledge concerning the research question. Also, the validity of the methodology is always justified by the review of literature. Secondly, it is a continuous process throughout the research process. A quarter to one-third of the total time devoted to the research is usually spent on doing the literature review (Coughman, 1995). It is started at the very beginning of the research until the paper is written completely.

Nursing industry is growing rapidly in the developed world nowadays. There is a growth trend towards professional and evidence-based nursing care (Burns & Grove, 2005). Research-based practice is essential to improve effectiveness and efficiency of existing nursing care (Barker, 2009). Literature review is vital to the profession's development as it gives evidence to researches that help to develop professional and evidence-based nursing care. In this chapter, both the importance of literature review as a continuous process and the practical ways to write it systematically will be discussed.

This chapter consists of six sections: a) Importance of literature review; b) Sources of nursing knowledge; c) Identification of relevant nursing literatures; d) Critical appraisal of nursing literatures; e) Combining the literature evidences and f) Presenting nursing literature review.

# Importance of Literature Review

The primary goal of doing a literature review is to develop a concrete base of knowledge in order to facilitate construction of the research (Wood & Haber, 2002). When the knowledge is reviewed, researchers will find out what has already been known and what has not been discovered yet. In this way, the review of literature gives researchers insight and knowledge necessary to develop research. It reveals the knowledge gap that needs to be explored. Meanwhile, researchers will know what has been discovered (Polit, Beck & Hungler, 2001). Duplication of researches that have previously been done can be avoided as a result.

When researchers have not identified the research question, literature review is good to give an overview of the research area (Pam & Goodman, 2009). One can get familiar with the research area by reading articles having similar research problems. The review of literature composed by researchers working on the similar research area is a good source of knowledge as it is usually brief and clear. The overview of the research area can be acquired systematically. The moment researchers get more and more familiar with the research area, they will be clear what the knowledge gap among the potential research area is. Studying research questions composed by other researchers will give insight and experience to construct a precise research question (Fain, 2009). By observing others research questions, researchers will learn to construct research questions broad enough to cover the research idea and narrow enough to include the specific knowledge.

Researchers can gain insights to design an appropriate research method from review of literature (Houser, 2008). Research tools like questionnaires and some particular measuring techniques can be acquired from the literature review also. In this way, researchers can gain invaluable experience on how the research question can be tackled from the previous researchers.

In addition, literature review is important to the construction of research theory (Nieswiadomy, 2008). It is sometimes hard to relate theory to a research that is still in the head of a researcher. By reading works of other researchers, the application of theories to research topics can be seen. This helps to develop the theoretical framework that is essential for a researcher to construct a good study.

Besides acquiring knowledge and facilitating the development of a study, literature review has important purpose that is not research related. It is worth mentioning that literature review has an important role in developing nursing interventions and policies in the clinical setting.

## Sources of Nursing Knowledge

Accessing relevant sources of information is important to the review of literature. Nursing books and journals are always included in the literature review of nursing researches. However, as books take a longer period of time to publish compared to journals, journals are preferred to demonstrate the latest knowledge of researches done (Thody, 2006). Some information in the World Wide Web is included in the literature also. But it has to be used with care as a lot of information in the World Wide Web may not be reliable

(Wolfe, 2000). I would suggest only sources from the formal and official websites like websites hosted by government and official authority should be included.

Most nursing journals can be found from the electronic database provided by the libraries of the universities and schools nowadays. However, some of the data retrieving systems are quite complicated (Langford, 2001). Techniques to facilitate searching may be required to in a certain level. It is recommended that a research novice should go to the library and consult an experienced reference librarian. The librarian will help in identifying the correct electronic database for the corresponding research and improving the information searching skill of researchers who have not used the specific data retrieving system before. In addition, researchers should spend sufficient time becoming familiarized with the data retrieving system that has been recommended by the librarian.

When acquiring information from different kinds of sources, it is important to differentiate between primary sources and secondary sources (Hott, Budin & Elizabeth, 1999). Primary sources of nursing journals contain concept, idea or study accomplished by the journal's author. Secondary sources of nursing journals are referred to as journals written by people reviewing the content of the primary source of journals. Secondary sources should not be used extensively in literature review because the idea in the primary source will be closest to the original author's perspective (Speedy, Daly & Jackson, 2006). However, a secondary source can give a different picture towards the same problem. Also, secondary sources of journals are usually written by professional nursing scholars, which give significant insights towards the problem area. As it is important to look at the research problem from diverse points of view, the use of secondary source in literature review is justified.

# Identify Relevant Nursing Literatures

Excessive material may be generated through the searching of the knowledge source. To identify the key works that needed to be included in the literature view of a research paper, it is essential to categorize what has been searched. At this stage, the details of the literature should not be focused upon. Skimming through books and abstract of journals is sufficient. Note taking is encouraged to highlight the central arguments and concepts made by each literature, which is helpful for the categorization (Aveyard, 2007). A list of concepts and theories should be able to identify each category. The interrelationship of theories in each category should be described (Ridley, 2008). The way how each theory or idea supports or contradicts each other should be figured out. A clear picture of the research area and the source of reference being retrieved will be generated as a result. After the organization of the relevant literatures, the key literatures that are most helpful to develop the research should be chosen. Researchers should give account to the concepts and theories included in the chosen literature. The concept in the key literatures being chosen should be able to support the idea and theory of the paper that is going to be written. Following, the key literatures that are being identified should be studied and described in detail.

# Critical Appraisal of Nursing Literatures

Critical appraisal of every paper that is being identified is essential to ensure the information provided is good in quality and relevant to the research question (Hek & Pam, 2006). In contrast to the preliminary step of identifying relevant nursing literatures, critical appraisal of literature requires detailed investigation of the paper being identified. At first glance, a paper may have point of views that strongly support the research question. When studying it in detail, the corresponding research method or data collecting method employed may not be appropriate.

First of all, a paper selected should be reviewed to determine whether it is written systematically (Lester, 2002). Details of information should be linked together in a systematic manner. By reading the research question, research method and data analyzing method, researchers can determine whether a paper is written systematically. The research question should be clearly structured. Rationale of the undertaking of the study should be sound. Meanwhile, the research method and the way to analyze data collected should be undertaken and described in an orderly fashion.

It is important to review the sample size and sampling method of the literature. In quantitative research in nursing, a large sample size can better reflect the reality (Levin, Fox & Forde, 2006). In some special occasions, small sample size is employed. Methods to determine sample in order to reflect reality should be stated clearly in the paper. Power calculation is usually employed to serve this purpose (Portney & Watkins, 2000). For the sampling method, probability sampling is used to make sure that the samples are not biased. However, nonprobability sampling is used also if a research wants to study a particular group of people. The reason of choosing a sampling method should be described in the paper. In quantitative research, statistical tests are usually employed to analyze data. Reference of the statistical tests should be included. To know how well the statistics generalize to the corresponding population, confidence intervals are usually used in quantitative papers (Bruce, Pope & Stanistreet 2008). This is an essential tool to know the validity of the data analyzing method of nursing literature.

## Combining the Literature Evidences

After a critical appraisal of the important literatures that are found, the literature evidences to support the research question need to be brought together. The primary aim of this stage is to summarize all the findings of the literatures chosen. However, analyzing all the findings, finding out the differences and similarities and interpreting the findings in an integrative way is encouraged (Aveyard, 2007).

To summarize evidences found from the literature, a table should be constructed first of all. The table should list out name of authors, date of issue, aim of study, study method, findings, strengths and limitations of all literatures found in an orderly way. This process is actually a simplified way of meta-study (Paterson, 2001). The purpose of the table is to give a clear picture of the content of the literatures found. It can facilitate the compare and contrast aspect of the literatures. As strengths and limitations of all literatures are clearly understood, construction of literature review becomes easy. For the papers that are similar in context, they can be sited together in literature review (Pyrczak & Bruce, 2003). For literatures that give strongest evidence to the research question, more weight is given when the literature review is written.

## Presenting Nursing Literature Review

After a long process of analyzing and summarizing literatures that are important to the research, the report of findings is going to be written. A number of guidelines concerning about writing a literature review are found in many nursing research textbooks. In the following, important features of a nursing literature are summarized to three main guidelines.

Firstly, literature review is usually the introduction of a nursing research paper (Lester, 2002). Literature review is always being used to introduce the research area. Instead of writing a personal point of view, researcher should cite literature that contains the same perspective.

Secondly, literature reviews should lead to the research question or theory purposely (Burns & Grove, 2009). For example, the literature review can give rationale of extending or improving a research that has been conducted. The knowledge gap described in literature review can also give reason for a pioneering research. The audience should be able to understand the research question, research theory and research purpose after reading the literature review. In view of this, the research hypothesis and question are stated at the last part of the literature review in most nursing journals.

Thirdly, the importance of a research should be clearly stated (Pyrczak & Bruce, 2003). Although researchers must be highly aware of the content of their own researches, readers may not be aware of their importance. Describing the importance of the research in the beginning part of paper is suggested. Some important factors that needed to be stressed include how the knowledge gap is being filled by the research and how the research being conducted is different from studies conducted in the previous time.

# Conclusion

Literature review is vital to the nursing profession's development as it gives evidence to researches that help to perfect nursing care. Literature review is important to cover knowledge that is important to develop a research question. Researchers can gain insights to design an appropriate research method from review of literature. Suitable research tools and research criteria can also be found from literature review. In addition, literature review is important to the construction of research theory. To conclude, there are a number of steps to achieve a quality literature review. Firstly, it is to access the sources of nursing knowledge. When acquiring information from different kinds of sources, it is important to differentiate between primary sources and secondary sources. Secondly, relevant nursing literatures should be identified; skimming through books and abstracts of journals is sufficient at this step. It follows the critical appraisal of nursing literatures. It requires detailed investigation of the paper being identified. Before the literature evidences are combined, a table summarizing all the literature findings should be constructed. It is used to give a clear picture of the content of the literatures. Finally, the nursing literature review can be presented effectively according to some guidelines suggested in the article.

## Author's Background

After finishing his first degree in Food and Nutritional Science, Lai Shiu Keung has been working as a music teacher for ten years. He discovered his interest in nursing after the leaving of his most beloved. (Email: sky_strings@yahoo.com)

## References

Aveyard, H. (2007). Doing a literature review in health and social care: a practical guide. New York: Open University Press.

Barker, A. M. (2009) Advanced Practice Nursing: Essential Knowledge for the Profession. Mississauga, Ontario: Jones and Bartlett Publishers.

Bruce, N., Pope, D., & Stanistreet, D. (2008). Quantitative Methods for Health Research. West Sussex: John Wiley & Sons.

Burns, N., & Grove, S. K. (2009). The practice of nursing research: appraisal, synthesis, and generation of evidence. St. Louis: Elsevier Saunders

Burns, N., & Grove, S. K. (2005). The practice of nursing research: conduct, critique, and utilization. St. Louis: Elsevier Saunders.

Couchman, W. (1995). Nursing and health-care research: a practical guide. London: Scutari Press.

Fain, J. A. (2009). Reading, understanding, and applying nursing research. Philadelphia: F. A. Davis Co.

Hek, G., & Pam, M. (2006). Making sense of research: an introduction for health and social care practitioners. California: Sage Publications.

Houser, J. (2008). Nursing research: reading, using, and creating evidence. Sudbury, Mass: Jones and Bartlett Publishers.

Hott, J. R., Budin, W. C., & Elizabeth, L. N. (1999). Notter's essentials of nursing research. New York: Springer Publishing Company.

Langford, R. W. (2001). Navigating the maze of nursing research: an interactive learning adventure. St. Louis: Mosby.

Lester, J. D. (2002). Writing research papers: a complete guide. New York: Longman.

Levin, J., Fox, J. A., & Forde, D. R. (2006). Elementary statistics in social research. Boston: Allyn & Bacon Pearson.

Nieswiadomy, R. M. (2008). Foundations of nursing research. N.J.: Prentice Hall.

Pam, M., & Goodman, M. (2009). Nursing research: an introduction. California: Sage Publications.

Paterson, B. L. (2001). Meta-study of qualitative health research: a practical guide to meta-analysis and meta-synthesis. California: Sage publications.

Polit, D. F., Beck, C. T., & Hungler, B. P. (2006). Essentials of nursing research: methods, appraisal, and utilization (6th edition). Philadelphia: Lippincott.

Portney, L. G., & Watkins, M. P. (2000). Foundations of clinical research: applications to practice. N.J.: Prentice Hall.

Pyrczak, F., & Bruce, R. R. (2003). Writing empirical research reports: a basic guide for students of the social and behavioral sciences. California: Pyrczak Publishing.

Ridley, D. (2008). The literature review: a step-by-step guide for students. California: Sage Publications.

Speedy, S., Daly, J., & Jackson, D. (2006). Contexts of nursing: an introduction. NSW: Elsevier Australia.

Thody, A. (2006). Writing and presenting research. California: Sage Publications. Wolfe, C. R. (2000). Learning and teaching on the World Wide Web. San Diego: Academic Press.

Wood, G. L., & Haber, J. (2002). Nursing research: methods, critical appraisal, and utilization. St. Louis: Mosby.

In: Clinical Research Issues in Nursing    ISBN: 978-1-61668-937-7
Editor: Z. C. Y. Chan, pp.43-53    © 2010 Nova Science Publishers, Inc.

*Chapter V*

# Research Was Not Done in One Day—Successful Literature Review Writing

*Franklin C. H. Man and*
*Zenobia C. Y. Chan*
The Hong Kong Polytechnic University, China

## Abstract

Literature review plays a paramount role in nursing research that can inspire new research ideas and help to lay the foundation for studies. However, it involves a huge amount of academic readings and requires certain skills on deciding on a focus topic and evaluating and organizing those findings. It is in no doubt a harsh task for the novice of research. This chapter is going to discuss the framework and the process of conducting a literature review. It provides readers with a background for understanding the importance of a literature review and what attention areas should be paid to while conducting it. After reading, this chapter will help readers to have a grip on literature review, relate the steps of a systemic search strategy for a research topic, and critically appraise the research articles.

# Introduction

When writing an article or essay, an introduction is substantial. It precisely and concisely expatiates the motivation and explicates the purpose. Readers can know about the main theme of the article and the mind of the author by reading it. In other words, it is a refined paragraph to introduce the scope of research and provides a fundamental background for the researcher discussion, and it is deemed as one of the most difficult parts of an article by many people, especially to those novices in academic writing who need to express the understanding of researcher in that particular research topic.

A part of it, called Literature Review, further illustrates the background and incentive in order to express how the researcher familiarizes with the relevant topic and to reveal the correlation among previous researches. It presents an overview of the relevant literature, brings out points that are important for the research, and indicates the importance of why a research is being conducted. As the role of the literature review is important, this chapter is going to discuss the purpose and process in conducting a literature review of a research paper in the interest of transcendent research writing.

# Purpose of Literature Review

The literature review is the part of the research where there is extensive reference to related research and theory in nursing. It shows the engagement, understanding and response of a researcher to the research questions. Literature reviewing and writing is an ongoing process that begins when scrabbling up the first article related to the research topic and continues until the day you finish the dissertation. It also refers to creating a review that appears in the research paper. It may have many purposes, and some additional points of view from other authors are given below to show the varying emphases that different study guides put on its role and purpose.

Boswell & Cannon lay out several points that a good review should include. Importance of the research, knowledge gap, theoretical frameworks, conceptual models, research designs and methodologies should be identified in the review (Boswell, C. & Cannon, S., 2007). They aim to provide examples for resolving problems, provide evidence for supporting hypotheses, and provide a context for interpreting the findings.

Grix also suggested that seven points should be included in a good research. A good review should *"focus and clarify the research problem*, expose you to demonstrate a familiarity with the topic area, highlight the key concepts and terms, summarize the accumulated knowledge of the topic area, identify gap of knowledge among literatures, contextualize existing knowledge base, and make you an expert in the field as part of personal academic development"(Grix, 2004). These help you to understand the purpose of writing literature review much more.

Some scholars (Saks, Williams, Hancock & Pringle, 2000, 30) indicate that literature review should *"provide an up-to-date picture of the research area of interest and show which areas have been investigated and the results obtained, identify methods of investigation that could be used in further research, give indications of problems that might be encountered and possible solutions, reveal common findings among studies, reveal inconsistencies between studies, identify factors not previously considered, and provide suggestions for further research."*.

Other book authors like LoBiondo-Wood, G. & Haber, J. suggest that reviews *"serve as a sounding board to estimate the potential for success of the proposed"* (LoBiondo-Wood, 1986, 62-64). The view also establishes a conceptual framework of nursing research by demonstrating the familiarity of all viewpoints and distinguishing between others scholars and own views. It inspires the researcher to determine which methods are used when exploring the topic area.

From the above citations, we can see that the literature review serves many different purposes and entails a wide variety of activities. I try to summarize the differences in the characteristics of a literature review. The literature review is a written, analytic summary of research findings on a topic of interest. It identifies a research problem and how it can be studied and helps clarify and determine the importance of a research problem; it identifies theoretical frameworks and conceptual models for organizing and conducting research studies. It also identifies what is known about a problem and identifies gaps in a particular area of knowledge. It is going to provide examples based on document studies for resolving a nursing issue and evidence that a problem is of importance. Last but not least, it provides a context for interpretation, comparison, and critique of study findings.

# Process of a Literature Review

Literature review often occurs early during the research process. In the very beginning, the researcher has a curiosity about something observed in practice. Then the idea is translated into a research question. A mass review of literature happens to see where the problem has occurred and construct the theoretical framework for how the study will structured, shortly thereafter to answer the research question. Literature review on a topic can provide an academically enriching experience only if it is done properly. Writing it is developmental, with each of the four steps (Ridley, 2008) leading to the next: Select a topic, Search the literature, Critique the literature and Write the review.

# Select a Research Topic

The first step in conducting a literature review is brainstorming about an idea or an area of interest. A specific focus and vantage of an interest in a practical problem is guiding your research topic towards success. That interest must move from everyday language into ideas that form a researchable topic. This topic must be stated as a well-defined question accessible to a specific academic discipline. However, selecting a suitable interest for research is critical to the success of the research. It usually begins with personal reflection and mainly comes from experience. Clinical settings provide the context for these experiences and provide fruitful opportunities for the discovery of issues leading to research topic. Research may introspectively uncover personal issues about their professional experiences. If one's own issue does not come to mind, other avenues are available such as professional experience, suggestions from specialists, academic journals, and so on and so forth. Oftentimes, the conclusion of an article is the location for suggestions of research ideas that provide another avenue that can inspire the idea of interest.

The research questions should be in a searchable format. How can we formulate the questions into searchable format? The PICO model could help to build the questions (Hickson, 2008; Gerrish, K. & Lacey, A., 2006). P means problem or patient. It states the target group of interest or points out the phenomenon of which is going to be investigated. I means intervention or exposure. C means comparison of intervention. O means Outcomes after interventions.

An example is stated as the following research question: "Do diet modifications improve blood glucose level in patients with diabetes mellitus compared to insulin therapy?" P: Patient with DM; I: Diet modification; C: Insulin therapy & O: Blood glucose level. PICO works well for questions about health care interventions. Once the four elements to the question have been identified, the next step is to make a list of all the words and phrases needed to search for each PICO elements. SPICE model (Oman, Krugman, & Fink, 2003) is a useful alternative to the PICO model for questions that relate to qualitative methodologies or the social sciences. Working in the same way as PICO, this model breaks a question down into Setting, Perspective, Intervention, Comparison and Evaluation. Using the above research question as example, S: Insulin clinic and complications assessment and education clinic; P: Patient with DM; I: Diet modification; C: Insulin therapy and E: Blood glucose level. This model helps to produce a more accurate set of results and to produce a useful list of terms for searching.

# Search the Literature

After selecting a potential issue for research, the next step is to search and to review possible data for the topic. Full ranges of literature that come from a variety of sources are available to support research and our writing. They are simply distinguished as primary sources and secondary sources (Hoskins, 1998). Primary sources are the description of an investigation or findings written by the researcher. For example, a study (Sovie, M. D. & Jawad, A. F., 2001) following the Donabedian Model indicates the correlation of hospital restructuring and its impact on outcomes. Secondary sources are the description of a study or a summary prepared by someone other than the original researcher. It typically fails to provide sufficient detail about the study and it is rarely possible to achieve complete objectivity in summarizing and reviewing written materials. They are seldom completely objective and typically fail to provide much detail about the studies (Denise et al., 2010). Possible data can be simply separated into seven forms (Gerrish & Lacey, 2006): Journals and journal articles, Theses, Reports, Government circulars, Conference proceedings, and Grey literature.

The first types of literature that comes to mind when thinking of a nursing research are journals and journal articles. These include all up-to-date contributed evidence to support clinical research such as opinion, editorials, letters, case studies and reports. Specialized knowledge is being delivered rather than generalized (Saks et al., 2000).

The second type is Thesis, followed by Reports. Thesis is the contribution of research degrees among bachelor's level with honors, master's and doctoral levels. They are considerably longer than most journal articles in order to provide an extensive record of a student research.

Reports are another type of resource that we can be use. However, they are often not included in major database and the quality may be variable as it seems to be the last resort when journals cannot be published (Gerrish et al., 2006). It is because they are subjective and do not address the central question of written reviews.

Government circulars are published by government departments and may yield useful facts and figures such as statistics and cost data.

Conference proceedings are presented by the speakers at a conference where they are presenting recent findings and providing up-to-date information. The last type of literature is Grey literatures, which are elusive and fugitive (Saks et al., 2000). They range from pamphlets and leaflets to governmental to health service documents.

Data can also be classified into different forms according to the content (Minichiello et al., 2004). Conceptual or theoretical knowledge base data includes theoretical literature, scholarly non-research literature and scholarly literature. Sources contain empirical data such as empirical literature, scientific literature, research literature, scholarly research science, research study, concept analysis and a study. Literature review article, analysis article and integrative review contain and evaluate a collection of research studies. Meta-analysis (Minichiello et al., 2004) is a special kind of literature that examines not just conceptually, but statistically, the methods and results of a collection of related research studies on a topic and provides both researcher and clinicians with valuable information about the state of the art.

Performing literature searches is a skill well worth acquiring and honing. It takes time to complete, and there are no shortcuts through this process. A badly organized search is likely to yield little relevant information and waste time. Some basic guidelines are provided here to help the search get started. In the very beginning of search, route of search should be distinguished first. Traditionally, manual search of books and periodicals library is reliable but time consuming. A computer search is rapid, easy and a less costly method for discovering relevant information while it has its drawbacks (Neuman, 2000). The materials on the internet provide a very wide range of information sources, but not all the materials are under quality control unlike standard academic publications (Houser, 2008). Some of the important and excellent researches are not available on the internet (Neuman, 2000). To tackle this problem, database search is one of the solutions. There are a number of computer-based searches of the literature that are appropriate to health care research such as MEDLINE, OVID and PSYCINFO. Literatures and articles of the database are much more reliable, as they have academic standards. Recording the results of a search are references to articles. For manual searches, there is no choice but to write out by hand every reference found. One useful way to do this is to use index cards. Enter each reference on a single card and store in a box like a card catalogue system of the library (LoBiondo-Wood, 1986). For each entry, include author, title, data, publisher, ISB number, pages referenced and the call number. This allows the references to be stored in some meaningful way at a later date. Another up-to-date suggestion is typing and computerizing all the references information into an electronic file. This simplifies the process and allows you to integrate information as you go along. Computerized searches will generate reference lists that can be transferred electronically onto a computer (Houser, 2008) and loaded into a database.

# Critique the Literature

The third step of conducting a literature review is evaluation and critique of what has been collected. This is to increase the effectiveness of the research. Only relevant works are mentioned and that excludes poor quality works and papers. Critical appraisal papers helps to determine how applicable the research is to daily life situations and whether it will help to ameliorate clinical practice of nursing (Hickson, 2008). However, there is no unitary method of critical appraisal. Some suggest a critical appraisal should be conducted from a logical perspective (Brockopp & Hastings-Tolsma, 2003) and should determine the question being asked and if the study design is appropriate and executed properly. Another method is recommended by the *Journal of the American Medical Association* guiding to develop the critically appraisal on medical literature (Gerrish, K. & Lacey, A., 2006). The methods focus on three basic areas: Message, Validity and Utility. Specific questions on those areas need to be asked for verifying the message feedback to clinical practice, if the findings are valid, and if the results are useful, respectively. Ultimate concern in a critical appraisal is the validity and the bias of a study result. A key principle of critical appraisal is that a good study usually provides enough information to help the researcher to judge that it is a good study. It is generally accepted that the components of the study that should be reviewed included Purpose of the study, Sample size and selection, Design of the study, Data collection procedures, Analysis of the data, and Conclusion. A good place to locate information for evaluation of the literature is in the discussion section, where the authors talk about the limitations of the study. Validity, Reliability and Applicability are the key principles of critical appraisal. Validity is checking whether there is bias or not; Reliability verifies the results from repeated measurements with limited variation. Applicability shows its implications for both current clinical practice and for future research. The above criterion are useful to distinguish the good literature reviews from thousands of hundreds of literatures.

## Write the Review

The literature review is not a list of references and article summaries. It is well-written information about a research topic that includes discussion, methodology, critique of findings, and gaps that require much more knowledge. Organization of the review is of paramount importance to make explicitly clear to the reader. It should include introduction, summary of the review, and summary of the current knowledge and should point out all contradictions and inconsistencies in the previous work (LoBiondo-Wood, 1986). Hypotheses and research objectives should be stated to indicate how credible it is, and make notes of gaps in the evidence. It is going to convince the reader that the information supports the need for the proposed study. As there are no formulae for literature review writing, different styles can be launched by the writer. However, there is some attention a researcher should pay in writing a review. A checklist of checklist of Dos and Don'ts for reviewing is suggested by Hart (Hart, 1998) as the following.
    *"Do....*

- Identify and discuss the relevant key landmark studies on the topic
- Include as much up-to-date material as possible
- Check the details, such as how names are spelled
- Try to be reflexive, examine your own bias and make it clear
- Critically evaluate the material and show your analyses
- Use extracts, illustrations and examples to justify your analyses and argument

- Be analytical, evaluative and critical and show this in your review
- Manage the information that your review produces: have a system for records management
- Make your review worth reading by making yourself clear, systematic and coherent; explain why the topic is interesting

*Don't....*

- Omit classic works and landmarks or discuss core ideas without proper reference
- Discuss outdated or only old materials
- Misspell names or get date of publications wrong
- Use jargon and discriminatory language to justify a parochial standpoint
- Produce a list of items, even if annotated; a list is not a review
- Accept any position at face value or believe everything that is written
- Only produce a description of the content of what you have read
- Drown in information by not keeping control and an accurate record of materials
- Make silly mistakes
- Be boring by using hackneyed jargon, pretentious language and only description."(Hart, 1998, p219)

# Conclusion

Conducting a literature review is a crucial part of the research process. The first task is to select a topic of interest to being investigated that narrows down the scope of searching. Second task is to search the literature for articles on the particular topic. This is aided by the use of range of tools such book examination in the library, and database on the internet. The collection of articles must then be evaluated for validity, reliability and applicability. Finally, the whole process should be documented in the form of a structured essay. This whole process requires certain skills, time and access to library facilities. However, a good review will provide an overview of the research already conducted, identify gaps or limitations in the research and act as a sounding board for future research ideas.

# Author's Background

Franklin Man chi-ho is a student of a brand-new pre-registered master's nursing program in Hong Kong and worked as assistant of anesthetist before joining the program. His decision to become a nurse germinated from his belief—People are not come to have servants, but to be a servant. He affirms his Attic faith after he graduated from his first degree. (Email: franklin_77@hotmail.com)

# References

Bell, J. (1999). Doing your research project: a guide for first-time researchers in education and social science (3rd ed.). Buckingham; Philadelphia: Open University Press, 90-98.

Boswell, C. & Cannon, S. (2007). Introduction to nursing research: incorporating evidence-based practice. Sudbury, Mass.: Jones and Bartlett Publishers. 97-120.

Brockopp, D. Y., & Hastings-Tolsma, M. T. (2003). Fundamentals of nursing research (3rd ed.). Boston: Jones and Bartlett, 110-119.

DeAngelis, C. (1990). An Introduction to clinical research. New York: Oxford University Press, 14-37.

Denise, F. Polit, D. F., & Beck, C. T. (2010). Essentials of nursing research: appraising evidence for nursing practice (7th ed.). Philadelphia, PA: Wolters Kluwer Health/Lippincott Williams & Wilkins, 170-193.

Feak, C. B., Swales, J. M. (2009). Telling a research story: writing a literature review. Ann Arbor: University of Michigan Press.

Gerrish, K. & Lacey, A. (2006). The research process in nursing (5th ed.). Oxford: Blackwell Pub.

Grix, J. (2004). The foundations of research. New York: Palgrave Macmillan, 35-56, 155-160.

Hansen, E. C. (2006). Successful qualitative health research: a practical introduction. New York: Open University Press, 23-35.

Hart, C. (1998). Doing a literature review: releasing the social science research imagination. London: Sage, 219.

Hek, G. & Moule, P. (2006). Making sense of research: an introduction for health and social care practitioners (3rd ed.). London; *Thousand Oaks, Calif.*: SAGE, 29-37.

Hickson, M. (2008). Research handbook for health care professionals. Chichester: Blackwell Pub, 23-45.

Hoskins, C. N. (1998). Developing research in nursing and health: quantitative qualitative methods. New York: Springer Pub. Co,10-18.

Houser, J. (2008). Nursing research: reading, using, and creating evidence. Sudbury, Mass.: Jones and Bartlett Publishers, 135-159.

Huff, A. S. (2009). Designing research for publication. *Thousand Oaks:* SAGE Publications.

Levin, P. (2005). Excellent dissertations!. Maidenhead: Open University Press, 26-33.

LoBiondo-Wood, G. & Haber, J. (1986). Nursing research: critical appraisal and utilization. St. Louis: C.V. *Mosby,* 61-70.

Machi, L.A. & McEvoy, B.T. (2009). The literature review: six steps to success. *Thousand Oaks,* Calif.: Corwin Press.

Minichiello, V., Sullivan, G., Greenwood, K., & Axford, R. (2004). Handbook of research methods for nursing and health science (2nd ed.). Frenchs Forest, N.S.W.: Prentice Education Australia, 10-14.

Neuman, W. L. (2000). Social research methods: qualitative and quantitative approaches (4th ed.). Boston: Allyn and Bacon, 444-479.

Oman, K. S., Krugman, M. E., & Fink, R. M. (2003). *Nursing research secrets.* Philadelphia: Hanley & Belfus, 25-43.

Pyrczak, F., & Bruce, R. R. (2007). Writing empirical research reports: a basic guide for students of the social and behavioral sciences (6th ed.). Glendale, Calif.: Pyrczak Pub, 45-59.

Ridley, D. (2008). The literature review: a step-by-step guide for students. London: SAGE.

Saks, M., Williams, M., Hancock, B., & Pringle, M. (2000). Developing research in primary care. Abingdon: *Radcliffe Medical,* 29-50.

Sovie, M. D. & Jawad, A. F. (2001). Hospital Restructuring and Its Impact on Outcomes. *Journal of Nursing Administration.* 31(12), 588-600.

In: Clinical Research Issues in Nursing        ISBN: 978-1-61668-937-7
Editor: Z. C. Y. Chan, pp.55-68        © 2010 Nova Science Publishers, Inc.

*Chapter VI*

# Ethnographic Research Study in Nursing Practice

*P. C. Chan[1] and Zenobia C. Y. Chan[1]*
[1] The Hong Kong Polytechnic University, China

## Abstract

This chapter is a review of ethnographic research. The aim of this paper is to have an understanding of ethnography, from historical review to clinical practice. Ethnography is a qualitative approach with origins in anthropology, which has been used in variety of nursing settings. In ethnography, researchers act as instruments, using participant observation and interviews to collect and analyze data in the fieldwork, meanwhile, they mainly focus on different cultural practices, cultural immersion and reflexivity. Ethnographers are directly involved within their study group, therefore their subjectivity may influence the objectivity of data. Transcultural nursing is considered necessary to apply in the clinical setting in order to gain new knowledge and improve patient care. In this chapter, the historical development and emergence in anthropology and nursing will be first overviewed. Then, the brief descriptions of ethnography will be introduced. The strengths, weaknesses and applications of using the ethnographic research will be discussed. Finally, the necessity of ethnography will be discussed as the conclusion.

# Introduction

Ethnography, a qualitative research method developed within the area of anthropology, has been increasingly applied into different fields such as psychology, sociology, education and even nursing. Ethnography is traditionally defined as the discovery and comprehensive description of the culture of a group of people, including understanding their behavior and views from group's own perspective. Buns (2005) puts that "ethnographic" stand for portrait of a people. It literally means "writing about people" (ethnos means people, race or cultural group, and graphy means writing or representing) (LeCompte & Preissle, 1993). This essay examines ethnography as a qualitative research method; it first identifies the historical development; it then states the overview, strength and weakness of ethnographic research; it ends this essay with the application in the clinical practice.

# Historical Review

Ethnography was developed about 100 years. It is the same as Anthropology, which is the oldest and popular qualitative research method that is still used nowadays. Regarding to the historical beginnings of ethnography, there is much debate on it. The early history of the social sciences found that it is difficult for the individuals to discover the nuances of people living together and sharing similar experiences. Therefore, they developed Ethnography. It is an old method, but it is as famous as sociologists recommended that qualitative research should be labeled as "ethnography" (Atkinson & Hammersley, 1994; Marvasti, 2004). Ethnoscience developed in the 1960s and was one of the research labels made from ethnography (Marvasti, 2004). Social scientists tried to increase the rigor of ethnography; as a result, ethnonursing has also derived from ethnography, which is particularly related to nursing phenomena.

# Culture, Ethnography, and Nursing

In the mid-1950s, nurses started showing interest in ethnography, because it acts as a source of information or as a research method, resulting in having better understanding of patients from diverse cultures. One of the major researchers, who was also the first nurse anthropologist, was Madeline Leininger; she wrote of her interest and culture and emerged with her working areas (child psychiatric mental health nurse) (Roper & Shapira, 2000). It can be said Leininger was the first to apply nursing science with the ethnographic approach. In addition, the most central concepts in "Culture" are also defined by Leininger. Therefore, she is regarded as one of the key developers of ethnonursing (Boyle, 1994). She formulated the qualitative ethnonursing research method in order to generate substantive and in-depth transcultural nursing knowledge. Leininger's objectives were to guide nurses to practice nursing with a cultural care and health focus and form a holistic picture of cultures and subcultures, in order to list out the cultural care values, meanings and action modes of each culture studied.

Ethnography in nursing studies was developed rapidly among the 20th century. From 1982 to mid-1995, there are more than 360 articles that were identified from an internet search to Nursing and Allied Health Literature under the term "ethnography." Now, ethnography's theoretical and methodological contributions are applied in diverse naturalistic settings by ethnographers from numerous disciplines, which include nursing and health professionals. Janice Roper and Jill Shapira, trained anthropologists, also worked on doing ethnography in a hospital setting, combining their experience, and then explaining what ethnography is, how it has evolved in nursing and how to use in the clinical setting (Roper & Shapira, 2000).

## Overview of Ethnography

Ethnography is a full or partial description of a group of people; ethno means folk and graphy means description. It can be interpreted as "A description of the folk" (Morse, 1994). Ethnographic research is not only referring to a specific qualitative research method, but it is used to describe the end product, which provides a mechanism for studying our own or other cultures. The principal methods used by ethnographers are participant observation, interviewing and examination of available documents.

There are two basic research approaches in anthropology: "emic" and etic." "Emic" is the insider's perspective, which includes the meanings and views of the people in the studied group. It also indicates considering questions and issues that are vital to insiders. (Fetterman, 1998). Regarding the "etic" perspective, it is the outsider's framework, the researcher's abstractions, or the scientific explanation. That refers to an external, social scientific view of reality (Fetterman, 1998). Ethnographers try to take on the emic and etic perspectives in data collection and analysis.

According to Muecke (1994), ethnography has been differentiated into different types. The first one is classical ethnography. Classical ethnography requires the study to "include both a description of behavior and demonstrate why and under what circumstances the behavior took place" (Morse & Field, 1995, p.154). Classical ethnography requires significant time in the field, continuous observation and making sense of behaviors (Speziale & Carpenter, 2003).

The second one is systematic ethnography. Systemic ethnography is "to define the structure of culture, rather than to describe a people and their social interaction, emotions, and materials" (Muecke, 1994, p.192). The difference between classical and systematic ethnography lies in scope. As the objectives of Classical ethnography are to describe everything about the culture, Systematic ethnography aims to focus on the structure of the culture—what organizes the ways of life of study group (Speziale & Carpenter, 2003).

The third one is interpretive ethnography, also called hermeneutic ethnography. The objectives of interpretive or hermeneutic ethnography are to "discover the meanings of observed social interactions" (Muecke, 1994, p.193). "Ethnography is quintessentially analytic and interpretive, rather than methodological" (Muecke, 1994, p.193). Interpretive ethnographers are focusing on the culture through analysis of inferences and implications found in behavior (Muecke, 1994).

The last one is critical ethnography. Critical ethnography is a special type of ethnography. It relies on critical theory (Muecke, 1994). It argues there is no originated culture; instead, the people and the researchers together create a cultural representation (Speziale & Carpenter, 2003).

Before going further, it is important that researchers define their positions before embarking on an ethnographic study. Leininger recognizes a specific approach in ethnonursing that allows nurses to "study explicit nursing phenomena from cross-cultural perspective." Besides, understanding the characteristics and stage of ethnography is necessary in conducting research.

The steps of conducting ethnographic research study can be divided into three stages, and they are pre-fieldwork, fieldwork and post fieldwork. The researchers begin by choosing the problem, group of people and field. Then researchers focus on the interested culture (field). After using different approaches to collect data, such as participant observation, the data will be analyzed and form an ethnography. When ethnographic research is conducted, data gathering must combine with data analysis. The two major processes are participant observation and ethnographic inquiry.

| Stages of Implementing an ethnographic research study | |
|---|---|
| Steps | Rationales |
| Pre-Fieldwork | |
| Choosing a people, field, problem<br>Searching the literature and gathering information on the people and the problem<br>Formulating a systematic plan of investigation<br>Making preparations | Identifying the culture to be studied<br>Identifying the significant variables within the culture<br>Literature review |
| Fieldwork Phase I | |
| Making contacts and gaining experience<br>Settling and establishing a role<br>Beginning to gather information and mapping out visible features of culture | Gaining entrance: Critical steps and sensitive in ethnographic studies |
| Fieldwork Phase II | |
| Working with informants<br>Identifying major themes<br>Focusing on gathering information on selected problem<br>Doing some sampling<br>Selecting additional techniques for further data collection | Cultural immersion<br>Acquiring informants: The researchers must have the support and confidence of these individuals to complete the research. |
| Fieldwork Phase III | |
| Continuing with participant observation— now raising more sensitive questions<br>Double-checking data<br>Obtaining large volumes of information | Gathering data (Elicitation procedures) |
| Post-Fieldwork | |
| Finalizing the analysis and findings<br>Writing up the study (selecting an audience, a voice, and data for presentation) | Description of the culture<br>Theory development |

Source: (Fain, 2004) & (Burns, 2005).

There are five fundamental characteristics in ethnographic research. Three of them are claimed by other qualitative methods; they are "Researcher as instruments," "Fieldwork" and "the cyclic nature of data collection and analysis." The other two could be exclusive to ethnography. They are "The focus on culture and cultural immersion" and "Reflexivity" (Speziale & Carpenter, 2003).

## 1. Researcher as Instruments

Ethnography provides the opportunity for researchers to conduct studies to meet the need for understanding the culture of certain group of people. Ethnographers as a research instrument aim to identify, interpret, and analyze the culture through study. They obtain information through observation and recording of cultural data. The role of participant-as-observer and observer-as-participant are suggested for ethnographers, but it should move back and forth among them. It is not recommended that they act as either participant or observer only, but both. Besides, Atikinson and Hammersley (1994) recommended that "participant observation is not a particular research technique but a mode of being in the world characteristics of researchers" (p. 249). The ethnographer becomes a part of the studied culture and feels what it is like for the people inside the situation (Atikinson and Hammersley, 1994). Ethnographers can access the "emic" view by collecting cultural group members' journals, records, or other cultural artifacts.

## 2. Fieldwork

All the ethnographic research happens in the field, which means researchers go to the location of the interested culture. An ethnographer physically situating oneself in the environs of the study culture is a fundamental characteristic of ethnographic work; they go to their homes, attend social activities, and assist in general daily life activities.

## 3. The Cyclic Nature of Data Collection and Analysis

In ethnographic research, different investigation arises from one researcher to others. Agar (1986) indicates that there is a problem, as no clear boundaries exist between the similarities and differences in human experience. Also, due to limited time and resources, the study couldn't finish by answering all questions. It should get and analyze data continuously.

## 4. Focus on Culture and Cultural Immersion

Ethnography is just a research method with the purpose of understanding the way of life of individual connects to, in which "Focus on the culture" is unique to ethnography. As Boyle (1994) mentioned, "Ethnography focuses on a group of people who have something in common" It is necessary that ethnographic researchers strive to discover and interpret the cultural meanings of the group. Unfortunately, culture is complex to define (Roper & Shapira, 2000). Culture is different in a behavioral perspective and cognitive perspective. In a behavioral perspective, it is the way of a group behaves, what it produces, or the way it functions (Roper & Shapira, 2000). For a cognitive perspective, "it is the ideas, beliefs and knowledge that are used by a group of people as they live their lives" (Roper & Shapira, 2000, p.3). According to Roper and Shapira, the application of the two perspectives will help to demonstrate "what people know and believe and what they do" (p.3).

Ethnography is an in-depth and lengthy participation of ethnographers. The researcher's participation has been called cultural immersion, which requires the researcher live among the people being studied. The participant observation would take months or even years. After the observation and the so-called participation, the nurse-researcher will draw conclusions on the culture based on his or her discoveries when collecting data.

## 5. Reflexivity

Reflexivity is the tension between "researcher as researcher and researcher as cultural member." It describes "the struggle between being the researcher and becoming a member of the culture. Because of the prolonged involvement as a researcher and participant in the group, it will extremely difficult to maintain a completely detached view." (Speziale & Carpenter, 2003, p. 158). This reflexivity has been discussed in many forums. Being intimately involved in the group, there is a struggle of objectivity in collecting and analyzing data, which is a unique characteristic of ethnography.

# Strengths and Weaknesses of Ethnography

Ethnography is holistic, where it contextualizes involved data, carries out observations and interview data; it is increasingly important in modern society. It is able to minimize the gap between different cultures, make people have further understanding of the meaning, value and practices of different customs, especially for those cultures that are distant. It is important to use ethnography in the qualitative research methods as there are several benefits that cannot be gained through other research methods. Enthonursing will be quoted as the example for discussion in this section.

## Strengths of Ethnography

As ethnography is a scientific study of human social phenomena and communities, it has in-depth understanding of culture among a group of people. The essence of ethnography determines what an observed behavior is or what ritual means in the context of the studied group. Ethnography is the description and interpretation of cultural patterns (Spexiale & Carpenter, 2003). Leininger mentioned that there are many other cultures in which such studies would provide a sound epistemological basis for culturally appropriate nursing practice. It may reveal embedded cultural values that were not obvious to the group, which is not a noticeable culture.

It gives voice to a culture to express their views; otherwise it might be ignored or difficult to hear from the outsiders. Thus, ethnography is frequently used for participation observation with interviews to collect data. The advantage of using participant observation is giving the opportunity to access information from the outsider's (etic) view, including interpretation.

Moreover, the usual practice of ethnographer is to publish books rather than journals as they prolong study and generate significant information. Therefore, they seldom only publish ethnography in a research journal to focus on only one facet of a larger study.

Ethnography can be used to study the previous unexplored areas, as the researcher can enter an unknown situation to observe, listen and document ideas and experiences. Ethnonursing leads to a high degree of realism; it allows nurses to study in a natural setting and view in the context what occurs in the real situation. Meanwhile, the major contributions of ethnonursing is to promote culturally specific care by collecting in-depth data, providing detailed accounts of nursing phenomena or experiences, within their contextual circumstances (Baillie, 1994). Changes are needed in the caring routines, like privacy considerations, room designs, and the way of services. It is beneficial to collect date from observation and interview rather than survey, as survey alone cannot represent the holistic picture.

## Weaknesses of Ethnography

Since ethnographic research studies involve natural setting and desire for discovering local person's point of view, the researcher should come together with local people and spend a very long period of time to live and observe them. Therefore, it may create several problems while conducting ethnography.

First, ethnography is a research method that is better to conduct by experienced researchers rather than the beginner; it is cumbersome and time consuming, as it involves a long-term period of time to collect and analyze the data. The expenses may be large so that the research may cost in an expensive way.

Ethnography may be inappropriate for analyzing complex environmental problems, especially when the climate is changing.

Additionally, the interaction between the ethnographer and the group of people is also important; nevertheless, several different problems may arise in between. As researcher will act as participant and observer in the field, thus the researcher's own subjectivity may influence the objectivity of the data. The presence of the observer may result in changes in the behavior of the people being studied. Data analysis will completely depend on the observer; therefore it is a risk when the researchers have not developed the ability to interpret results. Variations may also occur in the findings as the interpretations need to depend on the personality of researcher.

When applying ethnography in nursing, it may have the disruption on delivering nursing care. It seems that nurses may feel uncomfortable as their work is being judged or evaluated. Thus, it causes difficulty in collecting data. Besides, recording the field notes is another major difficulty. It is not convenience to write down the notes while giving care to patients, hence the accuracy of result may be affected during improper collecting methods.

Nurses may also experience role conflict when conducting ethnography, acting as participants, observers and primary caretakers; therefore, the observer may experience guilt at "observing" rather than "doing" (Baillie, 1995). These kinds of issues may cause role of conflicts, making nurses stressed and affecting the accuracy while doing ethnographic research (Baillie, 1995).

## Application of Ethnography in Clinical Setting

Nurses are "naturals" at ethnography. The ethnographic research methods can provide insights, which parallels exist between ethnography and nursing (Roper & Shapira, 2000). The techniques that were learned in nursing apply during the ethnographic process, including participant observation, asking questions, and considering information about the patient obtained from other sources.

Ethnography is increasingly used in the foreign countries. It has been applied flexibly in nursing practice. Nurse researchers use ethnography to study the culture of parish nursing (Tuck & Wallace, 2000), hospice (Wright, 2001), public health (Schulte, 2000), operating room practice (Graff, Roberts & Thornton, 1999), parenting of grandchildren (Haglund, 2000), and self-care practices of individuals with multiple chemical sensitivities. Within nursing, one of the major contributions of ethnography is to promote culturally specific care (Baillie, 1995). Application in the nursing practice is being important nowadays.

Nurse researchers have used the ethnographic methodology in diversity, such as studying a specific group of patients, like Preston studied the patients and their families that have done the cardiac surgery. The study indicated that the individual and family's health beliefs strongly influenced the response of health promotion advice. Therefore, it can select a group of patients with the extend observation in order to examine the details of their group's culture. Another study from Higgins, Joyce and Parker (2007) "Explore the immediate needs of the relatives of acutely ill older people during hospitalization." It is a descriptive qualitative approach using ethnography to collect and analyze all the data. The studied pointed to the need for education of stakeholders to focus on relatives as well as the older patient, improved assessment incorporating a whole of family approach on admission to hospital, which facilitated positive relationships between ward staff and families. (Higgins, Joyce, Parker, 2007).

Apart from studying the culture of patients, ethnography also can be used to examine a particular group of nurses or students in local hospital or nursing home. As Holland (1999) studied the nature of the transition period of student nurses becoming qualified nurses, he made use of ethnographic method with open-ended questionnaires and interviews to collect the data. It is a thematic analysis that can identify the dual role as students nurse and worker.

Meanwhile, it may focus on a ward or unit in the hospital setting to apply ethnonursing, like the Mcormack's study the nurse staffs' perceptions of the delivery method of nursing care in the practice of the general ward. The ward staffs make use of their diaries for three to five shifts of duty and interviewed them written in their diary. It applied the result for implementing of organizing nursing care within the ward setting.

Another example comes from the study of Jones (2002). It presents a large and ongoing study of an ethnography on dying in nursing homes. It conducts the study by participant observation, in-depth interviews and event analysis of the data in three nursing facilities. The results of this ethnographic are its lack of attention to cultural needs, cognitive status, inadequate staffing, and inappropriate communication between health care providers and nursing home people and their families as the main factors that influenced the experience of dying (Jones, 2002).

It is essential to have the transcultural nursing worldwide (Leininger, 1997), as there are increases in migrants to work such as Hong Kong; therefore, nurses should learn how to apply knowledge in the humanistic and scientific transcultural nursing practice. In the hospital setting, it is not even to provide services for the local people; it also needs to serve the foreigners, like the Hong Kong Sanatorium Hospital, where lots of foreigners will come to seek medical treatment. In addition, technology grows rapidly; many hospitals or nursing homes are making use of high-tech and electronic communications, so it transports the message and information more quickly between two hospitals and different countries. Furthermore, there is the increased demand of health personnel to view clients beyond the traditional "mind-body medical" perspective as a holistic multifactor transcultural care view (Leininger, 1997). Transcultural nurses' research study is needed to gain knowledge of the interrelationships and culture, and then deliver the quality of care.

However, ethnography is not being use commonly, for example in Taiwan. It has been found that ethnography has seldom been applied or discussed in the nursing literature from the search of different databases (Medline, CINAHL, Eric, PsycINFO, and the Index to Chinese Periodical Literature database.) There still exists many difficulties of ethnography that have been discussed previously, like it may disrupt the nursing care, and it is difficult to record during care. Role of conflict may occur when conducting ethnography, as it is not appropriate for nurses to ask naïve questions; it is difficult for them to have two identities (observer and primary caretaker). Being nurse ethnographers, they should plan their range of participation and observation cautiously, in order to maintain the scientific integrity of the study as well as the direct safety of patients (Baillie, 1995). Also, there exist difficulties in conducting long-term research; therefore, it still has a room of improvements applying ethnography locally.

## Conclusion

In conclusion, ethnography was developed by the discipline of anthropology for investigating the context of people's beliefs and practices, which is an inductive mode of qualitative research. It utilizes several collecting methods, like participant observation with interviews to gather and analyze all the data. Understanding the strength and weakness of this research method is essential for gaining the knowledge from ethnographic research, especially in the nursing setting. It is no doubt that it is quite challenging for the nurse using ethnography, like data analysis is time consuming and complex, extensive and in-depth data-collection procedures, etc. But many areas of nursing practice can benefit from these approaches, thus applying ethnography that understands the meaning of patients' behavior can enhance nursing judgments and improve nursing care.

## Author's Background

Chan Po Chu, Isabel, a year two student who is studying Master of Nursing in the Hong Kong Polytechnic University and the Hong Kong Sanatorium Hospital. (Email: Isabel_pochu@yahoo.com.hk)

## References

Agar, M. H. (1986). *Speaking of ethnography*. Newbury Park, CA: Sage.

Atkinson, P., & Hammersley, M. (1994). *Handbook of qualitative research.* Thousand Oaks, CA: Sage.

Baillie, L. (1995). Ethnography and nursing research: A critical appraisal. *Nurse Researcher, 3*(2), 5-21.

Barton, T. D. (2008). Understanding Practitioner Ethnography. *Nurse researcher, 15*(2), 7-18.

Bassett, C. (2001). *Implementing research in the clinical setting.* Philadelphia: Whurr.

Boyle, J.S. (1994). *Critical issues in qualitative research methods.* Thousand Oaks, CA: Sage.

Brayar, R. M., & Griffiths, J. M. (2003). *Practice development in community nursing: principles and processes.* New York: Arnold.

Burns, N., & Grove, S. K. (2005). *The Practice of nursing research: conduct, critique and utilization* (5th ed.). Missoui: Elsevier Saunders.

Crookes, P. A., & Davies, S. (2004). *Research into practice: essential skills for reading and applying research in nursing and health care* (2nd ed.). Philadelphia: Bailliere Tindall

Fain, J. A. (2004). *Reading, understanding, and applying nursing research* (2nd ed.). Philadelphia PA: F. A. Davis.

Fetterman, D. M. (1998) *Ethnography: Step by Step* (2nd ed.). London: Sage.

Graff, C., Roberts, K., & Thornton, K. (1999). An ethnographic study of differentiated practice in an operating room. *Journal of Professional Nursing*, 15(6), 364-371.

Haglund, K. (2000). Parenting a second time around: An ethnography of African American grandmothers parenting grandchildren due to parental cocaine abuse. *Journal of Family Nursing*, 6(2), 120-136.

Higgins, I., Joyce, T., & Parker, V. (2007). The immediate needs of relatives during the hospitalization of acutely III older relatives. *Contemporary Nurses*, 26 (2), 208-220.

Holland, K. (1999). A journey to becoming: The student nurse in transition. *Journal of Advanced Nursing*, 29(1), 229-236.

Johnson, B., & Christensen, L. (2000). *Educational research: quantitative and qualitative approaches.* MA: Allyn & Bacon.

Jones, J. K. (2002). The Experience of dying: an ethnographic nursing home study. *The gerontologist.* 42(3), 11-19.

LeCompte, M., & Preissle, J. (1993). *Ethnography and qualitative design in educational research.* London: Academic Press.

Leininger, M. (1997). Transcultural Nursing Research to Transform Nursing Education and Practice: 40 Years. *Journal of Nursing Scholarship*, 29(4), 341-347.

Macnee, C. L. (2004). *Understanding nursing research: reading and using research in practice.* Philadelphia PA: Lippincott Williams & Wilkins.

Marvasti, A. B. (2004). *Qualitative research in sociology.* Wiltshire: Sage.

McCormack, B. (2006). A case study identifying nursing staffs' perception of the delivery method of nursing care in practice on a particular ward. *Journal of advanced nursing,* 17(2), 187-197

Morse, J. M. (1994). *Critical issues in qualitative research methods.* California: Sage.

Morse, J. M., & Field, P.A. (1995). *Qualitative research methods for health professionals.* Thousand Oaks, CA: Sage.

Muecke, M. A. (1994). *Critical issues in qualitative research methods.* Thousand Oaks, CA: Sage.

Munhall, P. L. (2007). *Nursing research: a qualitative perspective* (4th ed.). MA: Jones and Bartlett.

Parse, R. R. (2001). *Qualitative inquiry: the path of sciencing.* MA: Jones and Bartlett.

Roper, J. M., & Shapira, J. (2000). *Ethnography in nursing research.* California: Sage.

Schulte, J. (2000). Finding ways to create conncetions among communites: Partal results of an ethnography of urban public health nurses. *Public Health Nursing*, 17(1), 3-10.

Speziale, S. H. J., & Carpenter, D. R. (2003) *Qualitative research in nursing: Advancing the humanistic imperative* (3rd ed.). Philadelphia PA: Lippincott Williams & Wilkins.

Tuck, I., & Wallace, D. (2000). Exploring parish nursing from an ethnographic perspective. *Journal of Transcultural Nursing*, 11(4), 290-299.

Wright, D. (2001). Hospice nursing: A specialty. *Cancer Nursing*, 24(1), 20-27.

In: Clinical Research Issues in Nursing    ISBN: 978-1-61668-937-7
Editor: Z. C. Y. Chan, pp.69-79    © 2010 Nova Science Publishers, Inc.

*Chapter VII*

# Grounded Theory in Nursing Research

## W. Y. Chin and Zenobia C. Y. Chan
The Hong Kong Polytechnic University, China

## Abstract

Grounded theory method has been widely used in different research disciplines, including nursing, sociology and psychology. However, little has been focused on discussing its development and the pros and cons of using this method. Therefore, the objectives of this chapter will focus on: 1) to explore the historical development of grounded theory; 2) to discuss the strengths and weaknesses of using Grounded Theory; and 3) to discuss the applicability of Grounded Theory to clinical nursing research in Hong Kong. By becoming familiar with the usage of grounded theory, clinical researchers are able to generate theories regarding to human health's promotion.

## Introduction

Grounded theory is a qualitative research method, and it generally refers to "the discovery of theory from data systematically obtained from social research" (Glaser & Strauss, 1967, p.2). The conceptual framework of this theory is largely based on the symbolic interactionism that emphasized the process of interaction among humans in shaping the human behaviors and social roles (Holloway & Wheeler, 1996).

This chapter consists of six parts: a) historical development of grounded theory; b) objectives of using grounded theory c) features of grounded theory d) strengths and weaknesses of grounded theory method; e) applications of grounded theory; and f) conclusion

# Historical Development of Grounded Theory

The classic grounded theory first emerged in 1960s, from two sociologists, Glaser and Strauss, when they collaborated on a study on the awareness of dying in hospital and how the hospital staff responded to the terminally ill patients (Charmaz, 2006). Despite the fact that they are trained in different backgrounds—Glaser was specialized in inductive, quantitative sociology and Strauss was specialized in symbolic interactionism—they have great achievements in shaping the foundation of grounded theory (Glaser, 1998).

In 1967, the publication of *The Discovery of Grounded Theory* was even the foremost book written by Glaser and Strauss to advocate the idea of discovering theories from research data rather than having a preconceived theory to deduce the testable hypotheses (Charmaz, 2006). However, in 1990, another version of grounded theory appeared in which Strauss and Corbin were the key figures. They have published a book called *Basics of Qualitative Research: Grounded Theory Procedures and Techniques*, intending to provide guidelines on how to conduct research by using grounded theory. They considered grounded theory as a method of theory verification rather than theory discovery (Charmaz, 2006).

To controvert, Glaser (1992) wrote another book called *Basics of Grounded Theory Analysis: Emergence vs. Forcing* to bring out the misconception of Strauss in interpreting the original concept of grounded theory. Glaser has restated that the products of grounded theory were theory and conceptual hypotheses, those testing and verification works should leave others who were interested to do so (Glaser, 1992). Though Glaser and Strauss have their own perception of grounded theory, their contributions to the development of grounded theory cannot be denied.

# Objectives of Grounded Theory

After reviewing the historical development of grounded theory, the objective for using this research method is to explore. The main objective of using grounded theory is to generate a formal theory by comparing and analyzing substantive schema under the process of theoretical sensitivity (Grbich, 2007). Parse (2001) has also mentioned the main purpose of using grounded theory method, which is to formulate a theory by gathering and analyzing the data systematically and by developing and verifying the hypotheses regarding the relationships between concepts.

As a result, grounded theory is the most suitable to use when there is little known about the areas that are going to be studied or when the theoretical perspective is not able to explain the existing situation (Munhall, 2007). The study of women's caring was an example given by Munhall (2007) to explain why grounded theory is used. She mentioned there was conflict in interpreting the conceptual ideas of women's caring of fulfillment, satisfaction, and life enhancement, and the clinical observations of women caring for family members is also unable to explain (Munhall, 2007). Therefore, there is a need to generate a new theory that is able to explain the situations. As grounded theory is strong at deriving a new theory, it is also appropriate to use this theory if researchers would like to view a situation from a new perspective even in a well-known situation (Glaser, 1994).

# Features of Grounded Theory

Grounded theory being a widely used qualitative research method, it has its own unique features that are different from other research methods. Firstly, grounded theory method is used to generate theory from data and it is different from quantitative research that started with some preconceived theories and hypotheses (Holloway & Wheeler, 1996). Secondly, it has its own evaluation criteria to judge the trustworthiness of grounded theory research study. The assessment criteria are that "the theory must be clear; the informants' social world must be so vivid that readers can almost literally see and hear its people; the research process must be detailed and must conform to the broad requirements of the constant comparative method" (Wells, 1995, p.34). Thirdly, constant comparison is used to identify the similarities and differences of data, and these data will then be categorized and coded to form some major concepts (Holloway & Wheeler, 1996). Fourthly, the collection of data and analysis will occur simultaneously (Beck & Polit, 2006).

In clinical research, grounded theory method has been actively used among the nurses (Field & Morse, 2002). One of the significant researches that related to clinical nursing practice is Fagerhaugh and Stauss's study (1997) regarding the pain management politics (Burns & Grove, 2005). The aims of this study are to find a new approach to the management of pain and to develop a theory concerning how people react and deal with pain in the hospital (Burns & Burns, 2005). Nurse researchers like Corbin (1987), Melia (1987), Morse (1991) and Smith (1992) were some of the representatives who used grounded theory in their researches. It is not surprising that nurse researchers would like to adopt this approach since grounded theory method is an orderly and systematic way to collect and analyze the data that corresponded to the nursing practice (Holloway & Wheeler, 1996).

# Strengths and Weaknesses of Grounded Theory Method

The following section will discuss the strengths and weaknesses of using grounded theory as a research method.

The ability to convert descriptive data into conceptual ideas can be one of the strengths of grounded theory method (Artinian, Cone & Giske, 2009). Grounded theory is the only qualitative research method that can generate theories from descriptive data. It is also corresponds to the main purpose of using grounded theory as proposed by Glaser and Strauss (1967), which is to develop theory from data systematically. It can be best illustrated by Dwyer, Lauder, Jamieson and William, (2008) in their study attempting to develop a theory to explain the problem that the part-time nurses are facing. Since the part-time nurses were unable to achieve their personal optimal nursing potential due to their motivators to work, employment hours, specialty, individual and organization factors, they will try to accommodate this problem by a process called "corrective juggling" (Dwyer et al., 2008). It is the process that intended to make adjustment to the difficulties and target on gaining a synergy and enhancing the professional practice (Dwyer et al., 2008). Therefore, by using the grounded theory, it allows the researchers to generate theory from the descriptive data.

Bias avoidance is another strength of using grounded theory method. It happens when researchers do not have any preconceived notions before data collection and analysis (Brown & Schmidt, 2009). As grounded theory does not require an extensive review of literature before the research is getting started, the researchers are assumed to be without having any preconceived ideas that can guide the study. Thus, it helps to minimize the bias in the research study.

Using grounded theory can also enable the researchers to maintain an open-minded perception towards the engaging inquiry (Berlin, 2004). Therefore, it aids to enhance the creativity in conceptual formation. As grounded theory is not attempted to adopt the previous taxonomies onto the new data, the theory derived is exactly what the researchers really wanted but not confined to what it is believed to do (Berlin, 2004). As a result, it can ensure a high degree of creativity.

Flexibility is also one of the strengths of using grounded theory that other qualitative methods do not possess, as it allows the theory to be modified at any time (Artinian et al., 2009). Brown & Schmidt (2009) have also stated that grounded theory is dynamic in nature and is subject to change when there is availability of new data. Since data gathering and analysis occur simultaneously, when there are new data that appear to be relevant for the development of theory, researchers can keep on modifying the theory according to the updated data.

Grounded theory method is also strong at studying those unfamiliar areas that little research has been done on. As Field and Morse (2002) mentioned, grounded theory has the utility for researchers to identify those unknown or unclear phenomena. Therefore, even the researchers want to conduct a research on unfamiliar areas, they can undoubtedly apply grounded theory to begin their studies and not be required to have extensive review on literatures beforehand.

Researchers themselves can also benefit from using grounded theory method as they can understand a study from knowing a little bit at the beginning to being an expert (Artinian et al., 2009). The process of analyzing descriptive data to conceptual formation can be exciting too because it can give researchers a sense of accomplishment after a new theory was formed.

On the contrary, problems can exist when using grounded theory method. Bias in forming the conceptual ideas can happen if the researchers are still preserving their preconceived ideas before the start of the research (Artinian et al., 2009). As Artinian et al. (2009) mentioned for one example, a student had a preconceived hypothesis that nurses would affect patient's manner in laboring. However, when she gave up this hypothesis, she realized that the nurse-patient relationship was actually influenced by other factors like patient characteristics or environmental setting (Artinian et al., 2009).

Uncertainty in obtaining the theoretical saturation is another possible weakness of using grounded theory method. Researchers may not be confident enough to determine when to stop the analysis and form the theory since a theory can emerge immediately after the start of data analysis (Allan, 2003). Therefore, researchers may need to try several times to achieve the theoretical saturation before they are confident enough to stop the analysis since they may be afraid of any new data that appears.

Using grounded theory as a research method is also time-consuming in reaching the data saturation. Dempsey and Dempsey (2002) have pointed out that saturation is attained when there no new categories of data are emerged and further collection of data is regarded as redundant. They also mentioned that incorrect data may be identified during the process of arranging the data into categories and thus revision is needed. For example, in Mottram's (2009) study, *Therapeutic relationships in day surgery: a grounded theory study*, the researcher has spent about two years obtaining the theoretical saturation. As a result, using grounded theory may take a long time to complete a research.

The requirement of theoretical sensitivity can also be a weakness when using the grounded theory. By definition, theoretical sensitivity is refers to "having insight into, and being able to give meaning to, the events and happenings in data" (Strauss & Corbin, 1998, p.46). As data itself do not generate concepts, it depends greatly on the extent to which the researches are read extensively enough to cultivate a theoretical sensitivity (Selden, 2005). Therefore, grounded theory method may not be suitable for inexperienced researchers as they may not have sensitivity enough to give meaning to data.

Another weakness of grounded theory maybe associated with the literature review. Owing to the fact that there is no extensive literature review before the data collection and analysis in grounded theory, researchers may not able to identify the missing link in knowledge and recognize the rationale for doing the research before the data analysis is completed. As Cutcliffe (2000) mentioned, the literature review section in grounded theory should be done before the collection of data and analysis because it can help the researchers to identify the knowledge gap or the rationale for doing the proposed research.

Confusion at the time of analyzing data can also be the possible weakness of using the grounded theory. As large amount of data is collected and analyzed at the same time, picking over so many words from each individual may lead to confusion and lose the focus (Allan, 2003). Accordingly, the researchers may feel disorientated when handling the mass of the descriptive data.

# Applications of Grounded Theory

Grounded theory is particularly useful for nursing research as it derived from a real-world experience and provided theoretically complete explanations about some specific phenomena (Andrews & Nathaniel, 2007). It is also beneficial to the knowledge development in nursing because based on the theory generated, the appropriate nursing interventions can be designed (Fain, 2009). As a result, through applying the grounded theory, nurses are able to act on the findings based on the theory developed.

In Hong Kong, grounded theory is uncommon to use in clinical nursing research and this may be related to the reasons like taking long time to collect and analyze data; researchers are not aimed at generating new theories or owning to their personal preferences. However, it does not mean that grounded theory cannot be applied in Hong Kong clinical nursing research since there are many grounded theory research papers found in the foreign countries regarding the clinical areas. The following will discuss how grounded theory can be applied in Hong Kong by referring to McCann and Baker's Australian study of how the community mental health nurse promotes health for the patients who are suffering from psychotic illness at an early stage (McCann & Baker, 2001).

Concerning the data collection method in McCann and Baker's study, in-depth interviews and non-participant observation with clients and nurses were used to collect the data since it allowed researchers to have diverse perspectives in seeking answers to the research questions (McCann & Clark, 2003). Questions that are asked in the interviews with nurses can be "What do you do to help clients who have had an acute psychotic illness to be mentally well and prevent relapse into their psychotic illness?" and "What can clients do to help themselves to be mentally well and prevent relapse into his/her psychotic illness?" (McCann & Clark, 2003, p.32). In Hong Kong, the nursing researchers are also able to apply the grounded theory because they have the ability to conduct an in-depth interview to collect the data.

After deciding on the collection method, grounded theory researchers are required to undergo the process of theoretical sensitivity. The sources for theoretical sensitivity can be from reading and the professional experience (Holloway & Wheeler, 1996). Therefore, the nursing researchers in Hong

Kong can use the grounded theory research method as they possessed the professional clinical experience. The theoretical sensitivity can also be gradually built up through extensive review of literatures in different disciplines.

Having theoretical sampling is one of the criteria to apply the grounded theory method, and it will continuously perform throughout the study. It is generally referred to "the process of data collection for generating theory, whereby the researcher jointly collects, codes, and analyzes data and then decides what data to collect next in order to develop the grounded theory" (Fain, 2004, p.271). In McCann's study (2003), there are sample inclusion criteria for nurses such as a registered nurse and employed as a mental health nurse. After initial data was collected and analyzed, further sampling was based on the emerged issue like nurses are generally supported to have right on prescribing medications (McCann & Clark, 2003). In order to have a different perspective, those nurses who opposed to have the right on prescribing drugs were interviewed again until other concepts emerged (McCann & Clark, 2003). Therefore, in Hong Kong, nursing researchers can also use the grounded theory method if they use the theoretical sampling instead of purposive sampling. It means that once the initial data have analyzed and new concepts appeared, those which could further explain the problem should be chosen as the continuous sampling (Holloway & Wheeler, 1996).

Throughout the study, coding and categorizing data is essential in grounded theory research. The coding process generally involves three steps and begins with an open coding. It is a process to conceptualize descriptive data into so-called concepts (Fain, 2004). For example, when the open coding are "getting them aligned" and "have a good relationship," it will then be given a conceptual label like "establishing a relationship" (McCann & Clark, 2003). The second step was to sort/list all the conceptual labels and the final step is to identify the core problem that the nurse participants experienced (McCann & Clark, 2003). For example, in McCann and Baker's study (2001), the nurses are facing the core problem of "uncertainty of direction," in which they feel uncertain when considering how to incorporate the promotion of health into the nursing care for the early psychotic illness patients (McCann & Clark, 2003). After constant comparative analysis and modification of categories, a substantive theory was emerged, which is to regain the state of patient's well- being, the nurses will take the adopting care provider-facilitator roles to interact with clients and others through the phase of engaging, advancing self-determination and developing linkages (McCann & Clark,

2003). In Hong Kong, if nursing researchers decided to use the grounded theory method, they can also follow these steps to develop a new theory, although it may take long time to generate the theory.

# Conclusion

In conclusion, to a large extent, grounded theory can be applied in Hong Kong clinical nursing research if the researchers can follow the analytic procedures step by step. The main drawback of this theory may be associated with the time to complete the whole study and thus researchers may not want to use this method. As using the grounded theory has many advantages as mentioned above, it is significance for the Hong Kong nursing researchers to use this method to generate new theories in order to improve the nursing care continuously in the future and to further study thos￼ ·nknown areas that may affect the human's health.

# Author's Background

Chin Wai Ying is a Master of Nursing student studying in the School of Nursing, The Hong Kong Polytechnic University. (Email: waiying_chin@yahoo.com.hk)

# References

Allan, G. (2003). A critique of using grounded theory as a research method. *Journal of Business Research Methods, 2* (1), 1-10.

Andrews, T. & Nathaniel, A. K. (2007). How Grounded Theory Can Improve Nursing Care Quality. *Journal of Nursing Care Quality, 22* (4), 350-357.

Artinian, B. M., Cone, P. H. & Griske, T. (2009). *Glaserian grounded theory in nursing research: trusting emergence,* New York: Springer Publishing Company.

Beck, C. T. & Polit, D. F. (2006). *Essentials of nursing research: methods, appraisal, and utilization (6th Edition).* Philadelphia: Lippincott Williams & Wilkins.

Berlin, L. N. (2004). *Grounded theory and its benefits for dialogue analysis.* International Association for Dialog Analysis 2004 Conference.

Brown, J. M., Schmidt A. & (2009). *Evidence-based practice for nurses: appraisal and application of research.* Sudbury: Jones and Bartlett Publishers.

Burns, N. & Grove, S. K. (2005). *The practice of nursing research: conduct, critique, and utilization (5th Edition).* St. Louis: Elsevier/Saunders.

Charmaz, K. (2006). *Constructing Grounded Theory: A Practical Guide Through Qualitative Analysis.* London: SAGE Publications.

Cutcliffe, J. R. (2000). Methodological issues in grounded theory. *Journal of Advanced Nursing, 31* (6), 1476-1484.

Dempsey, A. D. & Dempsey, P. A. (2000). *Using nursing research: process, critical evaluation, and utilization (5th Edition).* Philadelphia: Lippincott.

Dwyer, T., Lauder, W., Jamieson, L. N. & William, L.M. (2008). The 'realities' of part-time nursing: a grounded theory study. *Journal of Nursing Management, 16*, 883–892.

Fain, J. A. (2009). *Reading, understanding, and applying nursing research (Third Edition).* Philadelphia: F.A. Davis Co.

Field, P. A. & Morse, J. M. (2002). *Nursing research: the application of qualitative approaches (2nd Edition).* England: Nelson Thornes Ltd.

Glaser, B. G. (1998). *Doing grounded theory: issues and discussions.* California: Sociology Press.

Glaser, B. G. (1994). *More grounded theory methodology: a reader.* California: Sociology Press.

Glaser, B. G. (1992). *Basics of Grounded Theory Analysis: Emergence vs. Forcing.* California: Sociology Press.

Glaser, B. G. & Strauss, A. L. (1967). *The Discovery of Grounded Theory: strategies for qualitative research.* New York: Aldine Publishing Company.

Grbich, C. (2007). *Qualitative data analysis: an introduction.* London: SAGE.

Holloway, I. & Wheeler, S. (1996). *Qualitative research for nurses.* Oxford: Blackwell Science.

Mccann, T. V. & Clark, E. (2003). Grounded theory in nursing research: Part 3—Application. *Nurse Researcher, 11* (2), 29-39.

Mccann, T. V. & Baker, H. (2001). Mutual relating: developing interpersonal relationships in the community. *Journal of Advanced Nursing, 34* (4), 530-537.

Mottram, A. (2009). Therapeutic relationships in day surgery: a grounded theory study. *Journal of Clinical Nursing, 18* (20), 2830-2837.

Munhall, P. L. (2007). *Nursing research: a qualitative perspective (4th Edition)*. Sudbury: Jones and Bartlett.

Parse, R. R. (2001). *Qualitative inquiry: the path of sciencing*. Boston: Jones and Bartlett Publishers.

Selden, L. (2005). On Grounded Theory—with some malice. *Journal of Documentation, 61* (1), 114-129.

Strauss, A. & Corbin, J. (1998). *Basics of qualitative research: techniques and procedures for developing grounded theory (2nd Edition)*. California: Sage Publications.

Wells, K. (1995). The strategy of grounded theory: Possibilities and problems. *Social Work Research, 19* (1), 33-37.

In: Clinical Research Issues in Nursing
Editor: Z. C. Y. Chan, pp.81-90

ISBN: 978-1-61668-937-7
© 2010 Nova Science Publishers, Inc.

*Chapter VIII*

# Experimental Research in Nursing

## *W. H. Leung[1] and Zenobia C. Y. Chan*
The Hong Kong Polytechnic University, China

## Abstract

Science gives people feeling that impractical experiment is a by-product of science that is just written theories and wasting of money. In the following chapter, we would like to demonstrate how experiments can practically support our clinical practice and our daily lives, also the evidence-based outcomes can be the foundation of our professional nursing system. We will explain the purpose of quantitative research and the method of dominant usage of experimental quantitative research, discussing the pros and cons of the method, and finally demonstrate the implication to nursing in HK evidenced by historical revolution and phenomenon. In conclusion, positive and valuable attitudes towards experimental research can be enhanced, and nurses can be encouraged to be actively contributed in our future research activities.

[1] Correspondence concerning this article should be addressed to W. H. Leung, Email: hhuen_jasmine@hotmail.com

# Background

Quantitative research is a kind of paradigm that is describing a list work orientating need to be accomplished, simply like an action plan (Powers & Knapp, 1995); it is specifically a scientific process of validating and refining existing knowledge, also generating new knowledge and theory (Burns & Grove, 2003). It also is called as positivist paradigm due to the usage of logical positivism. When we trace the historical development of positivist paradigm, we found that it was from the early of 19th-century philosophical position of positivism: The classification of philosophies is characterized under a series of positive evaluation of science and scientific methods (Lincoln & Guba, 1985). Thus, this brings us a concept of reality that objects or issues can be objectively measured and evaluated with independent relationship of any historical, social or cultural contexts (Doordan, 1998). Every matter can be decomposed based on the pre-existing theories, or there are new theories that can be formed from the objective data regardless subjective elements, example as the periodic table of the elements in the earth (Cooper, 1968).

The objective of quantitative research outcome is focused on independent, measurable, objective data: Reality is composed of numerous independent variables and processes; any of the variables or processes can be studied independently of each other (Lincoln & Guba, 1985). After the analysis of the outcomes with different variables, a cause-and–effect relationship among the variables can be established. Thus, through the analysis, the established relationship brings the solution to concrete problems, such as betting on cards, understanding biologic inheritance, and improving food processing. (Barash, Cullen, Stoeltin, 2006) The dominant method is randomized controlled trial (experimental design).

This chapter consists of three main parts; first, we are going to describe the elements of experimental research design; secondly, the discussion on the pros and cons of the experimental design method, and finally with the application of the experimental design on how that can be applied to the clinical research.

# Experimental Design

Randomized controlled trial is called a true experiment; it provides a framework for evaluating the cause-and-effect relationship among a set of independent and dependent variables (Portney & Watkins, 2009). Moreover, it also consists of the highest standard requirements among all research design and as the golden standard to judge all other designs (Trochim, 2000). That means the experimental design gives the strongest internal validity data, also it simply means that the result provides a strong causal or cause-effect interferences. Thus two propositions are being addressed that if a cause is implemented, then outcomes will be occurred; on the other hand, if the cause is not implemented, the outcome will not be occurred. With regard to managing the independent and dependent variables that eliminate the interference or to test the specific variable, there are three main components specifically involved in the experimental design: Manipulation – to manipulate the action of the independent variables; Control - to eliminate the influence of other possible variables beyond the independent variable and control group is set for baseline data for comparison; and Randomization - to randomly select subjects from the population, also it is for randomly assigning the samples to either experimental (intervention) or control groups.

Basically, there are three kinds of experimental design: Pretest-Posttest Control Group Design; Posttest-only control group design and factorial design.

Pretest-Posttest Control Group design is relatively straightforward randomized controlled trial by comparing differences in the outcomes between before and after the intervention. The two groups are formed by randomization to equate the groups on one or more characteristics, for example, the score obtained from different IQ levels (Whitley, 1996), firstly rank the IQ score in order, then take the highest two IQ level applicants separately to the control and experiment group, so the two groups also contain low to high IQ level applicants.

Posttest only control group design is similar to pretest-posttest previously discussed in that applicants are also randomly assigned to one of the two groups, but pretest is not necessary, only posttest exist for measuring the outcomes. Although a pretest can be used to assess or confirm whether the two groups were initially the same on the outcome of interest (as in pretest-posttest, control group designs), a pretest is likely unnecessary when randomization is used and large sampling size is used. In case with smaller samples, pretesting may be advisable to check on the equivalence of the groups (Campbell & Stanley, 1966). Moreover, when the pre-test is impractical or potentially reactive, then only the posttest design is implemented (Portney & Watkins, 2009). In some situations, such as regarding to the study of hospital cost and length of stay, the dependent variables can only be assessed following the treatment condition, thus Posttest-only-control group is used. This design also involves random assignment and comparison group, its internal validity is strong even without a pretest; but there is an assumption that groups are equivalent prior to treatment. Because there is no pretest score to document the results of that, the probability of truly balancing interpersonal characteristics is increased (Portney & Watkins, 2009).

Factorial design is a matrix of two or more independent variables, with independent groups of subjects randomly and which is randomly assigned to various combinations of level of the two variables (Portney & Watkins, 2009). Theoretically, the number of variables can be induced without boundary, but in practical study, the increase in the number of independent variables, the increased demand of the number of experimental groups, so larger sample size is needed. So normally the study involves two to three independent variables at most.

Factorial design is described by the number of factors; that means a two-factor design has two independent variables; three-factor design has three independent variables (Portney & Watkins, 2009). This design illustrates the major advantage that it is more realistic to the real life that the important information that cannot be obtained with one single-factor experiments and it can examine the interactions that greatly enhances the generalizability of results (Portney & Watkins, 2009). This approach can be more realistic and validity then pretest-posttest design and posttest-only design since the presence of consideration of the interactive relationship between variables that the real world exist; this can greatly decrease the difficulties of manipulate the isolated independent variable, which may not be as feasible as suggested.

From the above three sub-experimental designs, we don't have any preference on usage any kind of the methods, but there is a different usage depending on the purpose of the experiment and the nature of the independent variables, the scale of the research and the time you are available to conduct the research.

# Pros & Cons of the Experimental Design Method

There are some limitations for using quantitative method for collecting data. As explained above, quantitative data collection method is to quantify the data into numbers, and statistics, then to find the cause-and-effect relationship, by the procedure of answering the nursing questions about the experience of health and illness or other required some subjective and unique personal view or opinion may not also satisfy the requirements of nursing as a holistic and relational practice discipline. The reason behind this is that the quantification can transform information into data, numbers, statistics that can reflect the reality of our world, but on the other hand, its lack of projection of personal feelings, descriptive analysis (Abdellah & Levine, 1994). As a result, the controlled characteristics of experimental design can't eliminate and classify all the extraneous variables and to establish the high validity and reliability of data-collection outcomes, just can be probably done. On the other hand, due to its quantitative features, outcomes can be easily compared such as pain is subjective feature, but after we quantify into pain score 1-10, we can compare the analgesic effect after administered Panadol. Its implementation is relatively non-intrusive and its analysis does not normally require more advanced statistical procedures as it just compares the different outcomes by the presence of intervention; so that's support to be the dominant implementation method of quantitative research.

Randomization can eliminate the causal variables and make the control and experiment group similar in characteristics and level. It also helps to assure that the two groups (or conditions, raters, occasions, etc.) are comparable or equivalent in terms of characteristics that could affect any observed differences in posttest scores and reduce the bias that could have that influent the experimental result.

Pretest-Posttest control is considered as the scientific standard in clinical research for establishing cause-and-effect relationship, but in the reality, can the control condition really be feasible or ethical? For example, when comparing a "new" treatment with an "old" standard or alternative treatment, or Synthetic Designs: A New Form of True Experimental Design for Use in Information Systems Development (Lee & Whalen, 2007). Even though there is no traditional control group, the design also can provide experimental control because we can establish initial equivalence between groups formed by randomization. As said, there is a control-based experimental group, and we can set different experimental groups for different variables which are also under randomization. Then the time can be saved by using one control group for experiment, but on the other hand, the sampling size will be larger and the data analysis will be more cumbersome.

Experimental designs also are limited by narrow range of evaluation purposes they address. With a complex subject system, rarely can we control all the important variables that are likely to influence program outcomes, even with the best experimental design, or can the researcher necessarily be sure, without verification, that the implemented intervention was really different in important ways from the intervention of the comparison group(s), or that the implemented intervention produced the observed results. Being mindful of these issues, it is important for evaluators not to develop a false sense of security.

We believe that randomization is a significant character that can generalize the result, which minimizes the effect of bias and personal issues. As a nursing profession, we need to carry out our cares without any pre-judgment, the same cares that can be received with different age group with different background. In the following, we will explain how the experiment can be applied to our clinical research.

# Applications to Clinical Research in the Local Context

Clinical trial is one of the most common forms of experimental design. It examines the effect of interventions on patients. In the following, we will use Hong Kong as an illustration. In Hong Kong, there is a Clinical Trial Center, which is a nonprofit academic research organization of the University of Hong Kong for carrying out and enhancing the quality of clinical trials from variety of human clinical research such as endocrine, respiratory system and others. The Center also created a freely accessible online platform for public to access, for researchers to communicate, for interested parties to register (Clinical Trial Center, 2005). The primary purpose of a clinical trial is to advance therapy for future patients. Furthermore, a new perspective of clinical trial in 2002 to see how oncologists view the purpose of clinical trials shows cancer specialists disagree about this purpose. The study shows many doctors feel the main purpose of a clinical trial is to provide state-of-the-art treatment to patients considering trial participation, and many clinical trial participants feel that the goal of a clinical study is to benefit them rather than future patients (Dana-Farber Cancer Institute, 2002). Especially for some critical illness clients, they have used numbers of treatments, but finally the prognosis is still poor, so they will think the clinical trial will be a new hope for them.

Besides the medical view, being the role of health care provider, nurses are challenged to offer creative approaches to old and new health problems, designing new and innovative programs that make a difference in the health status. This can be done by integrating rapidly expanding knowledge about biological, behavioral and environmental influences on health into nursing practice. Nursing research provides a specialized scientific knowledge base that empowers the nursing profession to anticipate and meet these challenges and maintain our societal relevance. (LoBiondo-Wood & Haber, 2002)

There is continuous anti-microbial wars in Hong Kong, the penicillin resistant, Methicillin-resistant Staphylococcus aureus occurred, the SARS, H5N1, H1N1; we can see that there is a new revolution of the bacteria, which enhances the attack ability and increasing the challenge of health care provider. The high awareness of infection control within these ten years in Hong Kong, from control use of antibiotics, the hand washing, strict control usage of the humidifier, the hospital bed distant restriction, the isolation protocol, which we can see we got the data from clinical, then with proven our hypothesis through experiments such as use of antibiotics, hand-washing experiments, the percentage of the alcohol concentration, etc. then suggest the best interventions into practical and enhance our nursing quality, to lower the suffering of the clients, and enhance our weapons against the bacteria. By gathering all the information and data from experimental researches, a certain guideline can be established, such as the *Recommendations on Hospital Infection Control System* in Hong Kong for public hospitals published by the Center of Health Protection (Scientific Committee on Infection Control, 2005). By following the guidelines, the spread of H1N1 is optimum condition, not as serious as in America and Europe.

Reviewing the existing usage of the health care instruments is also another kind of implication, such as comparing the effectiveness of using a lipido-colloid dressing for patients with traumatic digital wounds in 2006 (Ma, Chan & Pang, 2006). The advancement of the instruments such as the initiation of tegaderm that provides a transparent, antimicrobial dressing used to cover and protect catheter sites and to secure devices to skin, a prospective, randomized, three-way clinical comparison of Novel, highly permeable, polyurethane dressing with 442 Swan-Ganz catheters (Maki, Stolz, & Wheele, 1994). All these instruments are assisting our health care quality, standard and outcomes.

The data of the research can form new theory or revise the existing theories. For example, in Nightingale's Environmental theory, she stated the relationship between the independent environmental variables and the health. (Kozier, Erb, Berman, & Snyder, 2008). Also the data can be gathered as surveillance evidence that support the related actions: there is a Surveillance & Epidemiology Branch in Center for Health Protection; they will conduct research and survey in variety of diseases annually, such as Behavioural Risk Factor Survey 2004-2008 (Surveillance and Epidemiology Branch, 2004-

2008), that we can take further action for the changing trend, and monitor the effectiveness of the interventions provided.

All the above continuous enhancement of nursing practice will increase the quality outcomes of nurses, the clients, organizations and nursing systems; finally it will gradually building our nursing professionalism as whole. Since there is a characteristic of evidence-based support behavior (Freidson, 1994), the experimental outcomes provide a rational and evidence-based data to support the theories and behaviors and revise in clinical practices. Everything can be rootly traced with strong supporting.

# Conclusion

Experiment brings benefits on nursing practices, clients, community, health care system, health care organizations, and finally benefits our quality of life—all these contributions make us clearly understand, experimental research is really related to our life, not just a group of scientists' effort. In this chapter, we have highlighted three main issues of experimental research design, as being a role of health care provider, we can actively contribute to our clinical experimental activities, which may not be as large scale as developing a new theory, but it can be a personal experimental research topic. Through the experimental activities, we can be more sensitive to identifying independent variables that enhance our critical thinking on our daily practice. Thus, our nursing standard can be greatly enhanced.

# Author's Background

Leung Wing Huen is a year two nursing student who is studying in the Master of Nursing program in the Hong Kong Polytechnic University. She got the Marketing degree from the National University of Ireland, Dublin, and worked in the marketing field for five years in Hong Kong before starting the study in the nursing field. The reason for the career shift is the professional development of caring. There was a reflection when working for years in the commercial world; people are working hard to develop their achievements, but normally neglecting their physical health and it is usually hard to maintain their healthy psychosocial relationships with family, so she thinks life can be more meaningful and purposeful. In nursing, besides learning of a lifelong caring skills, she can also be the center of influence to promote caring concept; she believes world can be more peaceful by involving more love and care.

# References

Abdellah, F., & Levine, E. (1994). *Preparing nursing research for the 21st century*. New York, NY: Springer.

Barash, P. G., Cullen, B. F., & Stoelting, R. K. (2006). *Clinical Anesthesia* (5th Ed.). Philadelphia, PA: Lippincott Williams & Wilkins.

Burns, N., & Grove, S. K. (2003). *Understanding Nursing Research* (3rd ed.). Philadelphia, PA: Saunders.

Campbell, D. T., & Stanley, J. C. (1966). *Experimental and quasi-experimental designs for research*. Chicago: Rand McNally College Pub. Co.

Clinical Trials Center (2005). All registered trial studies. Retrieved from http://www.hkclinicaltrials.com/ on 28 Jan 2010.

Cooper, D. G. (1968). *The periodic table* (4th ed.). London: Butterworths.

Dana-Farber Cancer Institute (2002). *Journal of the National Cancer Institute*, 94,1847-1853

Doordan, A. (1998). *Research survival guide*. Philadelphia, PA: Lippinocott-Raven.

Freidson, E. (1994). *Professionalism Reborn: Theory, Prophecy and Policy*. Cambridge: Polity Press, in association with Blackwell Publishers.

Kozier, B., Erb, G., Berman, A., & Snyder, S. (2008). *The Nature of Nursing, Fundamentals of Nursing: Concepts Process and Practice* (8th ed.). NJ: Prentice Hall.

Lee, E. S., & Whalen, T. (2007). Synthetic Designs: *A New Form of True Experimental Design for Use in Information Systems Development*. San Diego, CA, USA: ACM 978-1-59593-639-4/07/0006.

Lincolin, Y. S., & Guba, E. G. (1985). *Naturalistic inquiry. Beverly Hills*. CA: Sage.

LoBiondo-Wood, G., & Haber, J. (2002). *Nursing research:Methods, critical appraisal, and utilization* (5th edition). St. Louis, MO: Mosby.

Ma, K. K., Chan, M. F., & Pang, S. M. C. (2006). The effectiveness of using a lipido-colloid dressing for patients with traumatic digital wounds. *Clinical Nursing Research*, 15(2), 119-134.

Maki, D. G., Stolz, S. S., & Wheeler, S. (1994). A prospective, randomized trial of gauze and two polyurethane dressings for site care of pulmonary artery catheters: Implications for catheter management. *Critical Care Medicine*, 22(11), 1729-1737.

Portney, L. G., & Watkins, M. P. (2009). *Foundations of clinical research: applications to practice* (3rd ed.). Upper Saddle River, N.J.: Pearson/Prentice Hall.

Powers, B., & Knapp, T. (1995). *A dictionary of nursing theory and research* (2nd ed.). Thousand Oaks, CA: Sage.

Scientific Committee on Infection Control (2005). Recommendations on Hospital Infection Control System. CHP. Retrieved from http://www.chp.gov.hk/guideline_infection.asp?lang=en&id=346 on 28 Jan 2010.

Surveillance and Epidemiology Branch (2004-2008). Behavioural risk factors survey. Department of Health. Retrievced from http://www.chp.gov.hk/guideline1.asp?lang=en&id=29 on 28 Jan 2010.

Trochim, W. (2000). *The Research Methods Knowledge Base* (2nd ed.). Cincinnati, OH: Atomic Dog Publishing.

Whitley, B. E. (1996). *Principles of research in behavioral science*. Mountain View, CA: Mayfield.

In: Clinical Research Issues in Nursing　　　ISBN: 978-1-61668-937-7
Editor: Z. C. Y. Chan, pp.91-103　　　© 2010 Nova Science Publishers, Inc.

*Chapter IX*

# Revisiting of Questionnaires and Structured Interviews

*Joyce L.M. Lam and*
*Zenobia C. Y. Chan*
The Hong Kong Polytechnic University, China

## Abstract

Quantitative research is a formal, objective, and systematic approach in which data is generated in numerical form. This chapter focuses on the data collection methods regarding the quantitative research study. Although there are many specific and unique data collection methods for different kinds of quantitative research, only survey research, in which data is usually collected through questionnaires, and structured interviews are chosen to be the focus. Questionnaires can be administered via three ways; they are mail, internet, and directly administered. Structured interviews are usually administered by the use of telephone or face-to-face interviews. Both pros and cons of each data collection are discussed. It is concluded that the application of both questionnaires and structured interviews in Hong Kong clinical research setting are applicable. It is especially common for the novice researchers due to the ease of use of existing developed questionnaires with high reliability and validity. These methods should be continued to be adopted for the increasing demand of research conduction in Hong Kong.

# Introduction

Surveys are a popular method used to collect information from a large number of people. Polit, Beck and Hungler (2001) reviewed that surveys are deliberately designed to obtain data regarding the prevalence, distribution, and interrelationships of variables within a targeted population. In addition, people's actions, knowledge, intentions, attributes, behaviors, opinions and attitudes are valuable data sources that are collected and involved in the survey as well. To do so, the researchers require the respondents to complete questionnaires or structured interviews. Therefore this chapter consists of the following main sections: overview of questionnaires, overview of structured interviews and its application in nursing research.

# Overview of Questionnaires

Questionnaires are structured self-administered surveys. Respondents have to complete a series of a set questions post by the investigator. Usually, either spaces are provided for answers or numbers of fixed alternatives are offered in which the respondent makes a choice by checking or circling. According to Gliner, Morgan and Leech (2009), there are three basic ways to administer questionnaires. They are mailed questionnaires, internet questionnaires, and directly administered questionnaires.

## Mailed Questionnaires

Mailed questionnaires are delivered to the chosen respondents accompanied with a cover letter and a stamped, return addressed envelope. The associated names and addresses must be first assembled. For those who are unresponsive to the mailed questionnaires, a reminder post card or duplicate copies of the questionnaire are delivered to them again. However, if the respondents are not specifically identified, questionnaires should be mailed to all respondents again (Gillis & Jackson, 2004).

## Pros of Mailed Questionnaires

Mailed questionnaires are cost effective in reaching and contacting a large number of respondents compared with telephone or face-to-face interviews. It does not require hiring a person to administer the questionnaires. While less time is required to administer on the part of the investigator, collection of data can be completed within a short period of time relatively, usually a few weeks (Murphy-Black, 2006).

## Cons of Mailed Questionnaires

Low response rate is often the major problem attributed to the impersonality and lack of rapport with the investigator. Fain (2004) reviewed that a response rates that range from 30 percent to 60 percent are common for the majority of the studies, however, 60 percent to 80 percent are considered excellent. With a small number of returned questionnaires, it is possible that those who are unresponsive may answer the questionnaires differently; therefore, it is inappropriate to generalize the results of the study to the target population. Questions are limited in length and complexity as the respondents are not given the opportunity to seek clarification. Those who are less literate and disabled e.g., blind, are excluded as well, causing sampling bias (Gerrish & Lacey, 2006).

## Internet Questionnaires

Interne questionnaires are the latest methods and have gradually become one of the most commonly used types of method in distributing the questionnaires (Gliner, Morgan & Leech, 2009). Internet questionnaires, usually accompanied with an online survey program, are being set up on the internet. Multiples techniques are utilized in the selection of the participants e.g., existing group (e.g., course or clubs), email lists and list serves, etc. There are many advantages to using internet questionnaires.

## Pros of Internet Questionnaires

Respondents who have computers can access and complete the questionnaire at home without restrictions. This is time convenient and promotes anonymity (Ahern, 2005). From a cost perspective, it is cheaper in contacting the respondents via the internet than mailed questionnaires. Furthermore, the collected data can be transferred to a data file directly, which can minimize the possibility of data entry errors. However, there are disadvantages of using internet questionnaires (Hulley, Cummings, Browner, Grady, & Newman, 2007).

## Cons of Internet Questionnaires

Stommel and Wills (2004) reviewed that the major inclusive criteria of the sampling are that the respondents must have access to a computer, therefore sampling is completely attributed to if the target population has a computer or not. This can potentially contribute to severe sampling bias. In addition, the violation of the privacy in regarding the rights of holders of e-mail accounts has been upheld, hence, data collected are not anonymous or confidential (Dilman, 2007). The respondent tends to ignore or cease to complete the questionnaire if it is too long. Therefore, the questions are limited in length and complexity.

## Directly Administered Questionnaires

The directly administered questionnaire is usually administered to a group of people who are assembled in a certain place for a specific purpose. It can be a class, hospitals or community situations, or any setting where people can complete the questionnaires together simultaneously (Polit & Hungler, 1995).

## Pros (Advantages) of Directly Administered Questionnaires

The main advantage of this technique is that a high response rate is usually obtained, especially if the participants are expected to be in that location. Since the respondents are given the opportunity to interact with the investigator, there is comparatively less pressure created, so it is possible that the majority of the potential respondents, 90 to 100 percent, are willing to complete the questionnaire (Jackson, 1999). Directly administered questionnaires also provide an opportunity for the researcher to clarify any possible misunderstandings about the questionnaires. There is a good example of how directly administered questionnaire is administered from the work of Landrum and Mulcock (2007). In this study, data are collected from the authors from students who enrolled in courses by the use of questionnaires. Students are then required to complete the questionnaires in the class. This methods is able to ensure a higher response rate than for mailed or internet questionnaires.

## Cons (Disadvantages) of Directly Administered Questionnaires

Directly administered questionnaires lack the probability sampling procedure with the fact that the selection of participants is usually done on the basis of convenience. Therefore, the data collected are not representative and cannot generalize to a larger population (Gillis & Jackson, 2004). Table 1, as followed, summarizes the advantages and disadvantages of mailed questionnaires, interview questionnaires and directly administered questionnaires as mentioned above.

# Overview of Structured Interview

Besides questionnaires, structured interviews are data collection methods that are commonly used in quantitative research (Hek, Judd, & Moule, 2002). The researcher has complete control over the content of the interview by using several strategies in standardizing the interview contents presented to the respondents (Burns & Grove, 2007).

Questions that are used to ask the respondents are previously designed and set by the researcher before the commencement of data collection. Therefore, questions that are asked will be exactly the same for all respondents and in exactly the same order. At the same time, they are given the same set of fixed alternatives for their responses. These fixed response alternatives are known as closed-ended questions and are usually used in quantitative research. It is how standardization can be achieved. It is likely that the interview may include a few open-ended items. If it is the case, open-ended questions are asked in exactly the same way for each respondent in the study.

**Table 1. advantages and disadvantages of mailed
questionnaires, internet questionnaires and directly
administered questionnaires**

|  | Advantages | Disadvantages |
|---|---|---|
| Mailed questionnaires | cheaper in reaching and contacting a large number of respondents do not require the hiring of person to administer the questionnaires data collection can completed within short period of time | low response rate due to impersonality and lack of rapport with the investigator limited in length and complexity less literate and disability are excluded inappropriate to generalize the results of the study to the target population |
| internet questionnaires | easy to access without restrictions cheaper in contacting the respondents via the internet than mail questionnaires time convenient promote anonymity minimize errors in data entry | severe sampling bias violation of privacy right, lack the anonymity and confidentiality limited in length and complexity respondents cease to complete the questionnaires if it is too long |
| Directly administered questionnaires | high response rate less pressure in cooperating with the researcher in group setting able to clarify misunderstanding | lack the probability sampling procedure not representative cannot generalize to some larger population |

As it is mentioned above, there are fixed response alternatives in the closed-ended questions. They can be simple yes or no or rather complex expressions of opinion. These high degrees of structure are made for the purpose of ensuring comparability of responses and to facilitate analysis (LoBiondo-Wood, Haber, 2006).

In some cases, the interviewer may try to facilitate the understanding of the set questions by elaborating more on the meaning or modifying the way in which the question is asked. However, a totally structured instrument requires the interviewer to ask the question precisely as it has been designed. According to Burke (2000), there are the two main types of interviews used in quantitative research and they are the telephone interviews and the face-to-face interviews.

## Telephone Interviews

Telephone interviews are very structured and brief (usually less than half an hour). This research technique is commonly used to obtain a quick, geographically diverse, or national sample. It can also be used for follow-up interviews with patients who are undergoing treatment for serious medical problems, such as cancer or heart disease (Stommel & Wills, 2004).

## Pros (Advantages) of Telephone Interviews

Without the necessity for the interviewer travelling to the respondents' location, telephone interviews reduce the cost of interviews drastically. Since there is no transportation time need to be included, less time is required for data collection. The interviewer can even use the time to do many more interviews in a day than would be possible if the interviewer had to travel to each respondent's home. It is more cost effective to gain access to people who have difficulties in arranging the interview appointment such as physicians or people who scattered in different regions or disabled individuals such as the blind (Gillis & Jackson, 2004). It is possible that the nature of the research topic may create a risk of respondents perceiving that they would be judged or they may have conflicting commitments; therefore, telephone interviews provide a sensitive platform for them to reject the interview and ensure they are not under any pressure to participate (Gerrish & Lacey, 2006).

## Cons (Disadvantages) of Telephone Interviews

The response rate may be adversely affected as the potential respondents of telephone interviews are restricted to those who have phones. Meanwhile, due to the increasing number of unlisted telephone numbers and screening technology for incoming calls, the accessibility to the respondents via telephone decreased (Dilman, 2000). And as there is increasing marketing promotion via the telephone, many of the potential respondents may not answer the phone. Telephone interviews lack the visual contacts, making it impossible for the interviewer to gauge the condition of the respondent and using visual clues to facilitate questioning; therefore, it minimizes the ability to obtain detailed information, misinformation and the emotional implications (Gerrish & Lacey, 2006). Telephone interviews are less well adapted to managing lengthy and complex response scales, for example a standard Likert response scale with five or more choices, such as "strongly disagree," "agree," "neutral," "agree," and "strongly agree." The interviewer has to repeat all these alternatives every single time when a new question is asked. This is not only tedious, but also annoying for both the interview and the respondent (Stommel & Wills, 2004).

## Face-to-Face Interviews

For face-to-face interviews, the set questions are read to the respondents. The interviewer is expected to read the questions, exactly as worded and record responses by pen or directly into the computer. This approach is usually used for closed questions.

## Pros (Advantages) of Face-to-Face Interviews

Because the respondent becomes known to the interviewer, substitution of other respondents for the desired or designated respondent is difficult (Fielding, 2003). Physical presence and visual contacts permit the interviewer to observe the respondents and collect additional clues. Unlike the telephone interview, face-to-face interview can be more suitable for complex interviews as mentioned previously. Interviewer is allowed to utilize visual aids such as a cue card that enables the interviewee to easily make choices directly from a list of multiple alternatives. The response rate tends to be high in face-to-face interviews as the respondents are generally less likely to refuse to talk to an interviewer than to ignore questionnaires, especially a mailed questionnaire. Misinterpretations of questions are avoided as the interviewer is present to determine whether questions have been misunderstood (Stommel & Wills, 2004).

## Cons (Disadvantages) of Face-to-Face Interviews

However, face-to-face structured interviews offer fewer opportunities for the interviewees to elaborate on their responses; therefore, data collected may be superficial and lacking anonymity. The cost of transportation for face-to-face interviews is expensive and time consuming; they are normally done when small sample size is required (Green & Thorogood, 2009). And as a sensitive research topic is involved, the interviewees may be embarrassed to answer questions such as risk-taking behavior, sexual dysfunction, urinary problems, etc. (Stommel & Wills, 2004). Table 2 summaries the advantages and disadvantages of both telephone and face-to-face interviews.

**Table 2. advantages and disadvantages of
telephone and face-to-face interviews**

|  | Advantages | Disadvantage |
|---|---|---|
| Telephone interview | no transportation required shortened data collection time lower cost less pressure to participants gain access to people who have difficulties in arranging the interview appointment | potential respondent restricted to those with phone advanced screening technology potential respondents avoid answering the phone lacks the visual contacts and visual clues to facilitate questioning not suitable for lengthy and complex response scales tedious and annoying |
| Face-to-face interview | substitution of other respondents is difficult physical presence and allows visual contacts able to observe and collect additional clues suitable for complex interviews as visual aids can be utilized, e.g., cue card higher response rate less prone to misinterpretation | data collected may be superficial expensive time consuming lack of anonymity not suitable for sensitive topics |

## Comparison between Questionnaires and Structured Interviews

Here we have discussed the different types of questionnaires and structured interviews; a brief comparison between the two methods will be discussed. Questionnaires require less cost than structured interviews as the cost of transportation to each respondents and the hiring of interviewers are excluded and hence, they reach a larger sample size among wider distances geographically. However, except the directly administered questionnaires in groups, both internet and mailed questionnaires lack the direct contact with the interviewers compared with structured interviews, the opportunities to clarify questions are less, and questions are limited in length and complexity but offer anonymity. Structured interviews allow the respondents to answer questions verbally; therefore, those who are less literate and disabled are included in the research study, and sampling is less biased. Table 3, as follows, provides a brief summary of the strengths and weaknesses for both questionnaires and structured interviews.

### Table 3. strengths and weaknesses of questionnaires and structured interviews

|  | strength | weakness |
|---|---|---|
| questionnaires | less cost<br>less time required<br>offer anonymity | larger sample size among wider distances geographically<br>limited in length and complexity<br>lack the opportunity for clarification |
| Structured interviews | questions can be more complex and in depth<br>offer changes for clarification<br>included those who are less literates and disabled<br>sampling is less biased | costly for transportation and hiring of interviewers<br>lack the anonymity and confidentiality |

# Application in Hong Kong Clinical Research

The application of both questionnaires and structured interviews in the research of Hong Kong are possible and will be discussed as follows. There are many existing developed questionnaires with high reliability and validity that can be used. Therefore, it is especially popular and used among the novice researcher as it is easier in conduct, control and formulate data analysis, and therefore less error will result. However, one should aware of the content in formulating the questions if the researchers want to develop their own questions. Questions should be relevant and enable the respondents to answer the questions and the use of language should be appropriate concerning the target population. Therefore, the willingness to respond will be enhanced if questions do not expose ignorance.

Both methods should be continued to be used and would never replace one another. This is very realistic in regarding the aging population in Hong Kong. It is inevitable that many more clinical researches are expected to be conducted in the future in regarding elderly. Therefore, questionnaires may not be applicable or the best options, but rather structured interviews, because they are less accustomed to writing or uncomfortable with writing or with low literacy skills. Therefore, both questionnaires and structured interviews are valuable data collection methods and should continually be utilized.

# Conclusion

This chapter examines questionnaires and structured interviews regarding survey research. Questionnaires can be distributed via the mail, internet, and directly administered, whereas a structured interview can be organized either by the use of telephone or by face-to-face interview. Both pros and cons of each data collection method are discussed and the applications of data collection methods in the Hong Kong clinical research are mentioned. Both methods are suitable for novice researchers as it is easier to conduct, collect and analyze the data. Nursing educators should equip their nursing students well in using these data collection methods. The nurse researchers, as well, should maximize the utilization of both methods.

# Author's Background

Lok Man Joyce Lam
In preserving high quality care, evidence-based practices would never be abandoned. Nurses should participate and conduct research rigorously and implement research findings in practice in promoting patients' well-being. Meanwhile, the conduction of research study is the fundamental building block in underpinning the profession of nursing.
(Email: joycemanman@hotmail.com)

# References

Ahern, N.R. (2005). Using the internet to conduct research. *Nurse researcher. Interviewing. 13*(2),55-70.

Burk, J. (2000). *Educational research: Quantitative and qualitative approach.* Boston: Allyn and Bacon.

Burns, N., & Grove, S.K. (2007). *Understanding nursing research: Building and evidence- based practice* (4th ed). St. Louis: Saunders Elsevier.

Dilman, D.A. (2000). *Mail and internet surveys: The total design method.* New York: Wiley.

Dilman, D.A. (2007). *Mail and internet surveys: The tailored design method* (2nd ed.). Thousand Oaks, CA: Sage.

Fain, J.A. (2004). *Reading, understanding, and applying nursing research: A test and workbook* (2nd ed.). Philadeplhia: F.A. Davis Company.

Fielding, N. (2003). *Interviewing.* Thousand Oaks. CA: Sage.

Gerrish, K., & Lacey, A. (2006). *The research process in nursing* (5th ed.). USA: Blackwell.

Gillis, A., & Kackson, W. (2004). *Research for nurses methods and interpretation.* Philadelphia: F.A. Davis Company.

Gliner, J. A, Morgan, G. A., & Leech, N.L. (2009). *Research methods in applied settings: An integrated approach to design and analysis* (2nd ed.). New York: Routledge.

Green, J., & Thorogood, N. (2009). *Qualitative methods for health research* (2nd ed.). London: Sage Publications.

Hek, G., Judd, M., & Moule, P. (2002). *Making sense of research: an introduction for health and social care practitioners* (2nd ed.). London: Continuum.

Hulley, S. B., Cummings, S. R., Browner, W. S., Grady, D. G., & Newman, T. B. (2007). *Designing clinical research (3rd ed.).* Philadelphia: Lippincott Williams & Wilkins.

Jackson, W. (1999). *Methods: Doing social research* (2nd ed.). Scarborough, Ont.: Prentice Hall (Canada).

LoBiondo-Wood, G., Haber, J. (2006). *Nursing research: Methods and critical appraisal for evidence-based practice* (6th ed.). Missouri: Mosby.

Landrum, R.E., & Mulcock, S.D. (2007). Use of pre- and post surveys to predict student outcomes. *Teaching of Psychology, 34,* 163-166.

Murphy-Black, T. (2006). Using questionnaires. In K.Gerrish & A.Lacey (5th ed.), *The research process in nursing* (pp. 367-382).Oxford: Blackwell Publishing.

Polit, D.F., Beck, C.T., & Hungler, B.P. (2001). *Essentials of nursing research: Methods, appraisal, and utilization* (5th ed.). Philadelphia: Lippincott.

Polit, D.F., & Hungler, B.P. (1995). *Nursing research: Principles and methods* (5th ed.). Philadelphia: J.B. Lippincott Company.

Stommel, M, & Wills, C.E. (2004). *Clinical research: Concepts and principles for advanced practice nurses*. Philadelphia: Lippincott Williams & Wilkins.

In: Clinical Research Issues in Nursing          ISBN: 978-1-61668-937-7
Editor: Z. C. Y. Chan, pp.105-118          © 2010 Nova Science Publishers, Inc.

*Chapter X*

# Observation Methods and Questionnaires in Nursing Research

## *W. Y. Tam and Zenobia C. Y. Chan*

The Hong Kong Polytechnic University, China

## Abstract

Quantitative research method is a deductive approach for the testing of hypothesis to investigate certain phenomena. It was used to study the relationship among quantifiable variables. The use of statistical instrument for data analysis is one of the characteristics of quantitative research. There are different types of quantitative research methods that can be used in the nursing studies. In this chapter, the observation methods and questionnaires will be discussed. This chapter consists of five sections including observation methods, questionnaires, comparison of observation methods and questionnaires, application in nursing research and conclusion.

## Observation Methods

Observation methods can be used in dealing with habits and other attributes that may be difficult to elicit by the use of survey instruments. It involves the description and analysis of behaviors. Observation can be divided into structured and unstructured ones (Dempsey & Dempsey, 2000). For the unstructured observation, behaviors are identified and observed in a descriptive manner. On the contrary, for the structured observation, specific parameters and standards are set before carrying out observation. Quantified results are obtained throughout the structured observation process. Therefore, structured observation methods are more commonly used in the quantitative research (Casey, 2006).

In the structured observation, the researcher needs to determine the time, system for obtaining accurate records and training of observers (Gerish & Lacey, 2006). Time sampling and event sampling methods can be used. Time sampling is a method with an identified universe of time with either systematic or random sampling design (Burns & Grove, 2007). Time sampling is usually more representative than event sampling. On the contrary, event sampling involves selecting only events or occurrence of a given class. Its advantages include: the inheriting of validity, continuity of behavior and capturing events of interest that are infrequent.

Categories and checklists are always be used for the structured observation. It is important to set the number of categories to be small, and to minimize the influence of the observer's inference to a moderate level by providing specific examples of behavior (Brockopp & Hastings-Tolsma, 2003). Checklists can be used for the observer to identify and record types and frequency of particular behaviors on the list. Rating scales can also be used in the observation checklist. The researcher then determines the frequencies of occurrence and counts the results. This provides a foundation for interpretations and conclusion about the certain specific behavior (Gillis & Jackson, 2002). Videotaping can be used to assist in recording the observations. It can capture complex behavior and make the capture of a scene permanent. It produces less disturbance to the scene by concealed camera than a human observer. However, it is necessary to obtain consent from the subjects when performing videotaping. Its disadvantage is that there is only one view of a situation, and it may thus give the observer a distorted impression (Lobiondo-Wood, Haber, Cameron & Sigh, 2009).

As the characteristics of observation methods mentioned above, we can suggest that the observation methods are well suited in many nursing research settings. Since the job nature and the training of a nurse is to watch the people's behaviors, it enables most of the nurses to become sensitive observers. Moreover, the observation methods can be more appropriate research tools when the subjects cannot adequately describe their behaviors (e.g., young children or the mentally ill patient), or in the study of the behaviors that are unaware (e.g., stress-induced behavior) or undesirable (e.g., hostile behavior), since there is a relatively high potential of bias in self-reporting method. In these situations, observational methods can be applied as unique and intelligent tools for measurement (Polit & Beck, 2006).

# Questionnaires

Questionnaires are commonly used to obtain people's opinions or attitudes (Jack & Clarke, 1998). Two types of questions that can be used when setting the questionnaire: open-ended questions and closed-ended questions. Open-ended questions give freedom for the respondents to express their answers. It is mainly used for the exploratory purpose. For close-ended questions, the researcher has predicted for the respondent's response and provided a set of fixed alternative formatted answers under each question. The parameters in close-ended question are measurable, quantified, classified, or categorized. It enables the uniformity of the responses and facilitates the data analysis. Therefore, close-ended question are more commonly used in quantitative research (Thom, 2007).

In the following, the qualities of a good (with high response rate and validity) questionnaire are discussed. Firstly, questions in the questionnaire should be precise and concise. Short items enable the respondent to read quickly and facilitate the yield of a high response rate. It is especially important when constructing questionnaire to the subjects who are physically or mentally compromised or who may tire easily. Larger fonts than the normal type can be used when the questionnaires are prepared to give to the elderly subjects. Generally, the optimal length of a questionnaire takes no longer than 20 minutes to complete. A lengthy questionnaire would discourage the people from participating in the study or make the respondent fatigued and fail to complete all the questions. However, if the questionnaire is too short, it may give people an impression that this questionnaire is unimportant and also result in a low response rate (McGibbon, 1997b; Meadows, 2003). Close-ended questions can be used to enhance the response rate for the respondent who is poorly motivated to formulate their own answers.

Items should be relevant to most of the potential respondents. Researcher should try to include all possible responses for the respondent when generating questionnaires. The item "others" can be added with a blank for the respondent to give supplementary information for the answer to enhance the inclusiveness of the data collection from the questionnaires. These measures can avoid the respondent being frustrated by encountering too many "not applicable" questions or being forced to select the "closest answer" when they found that their desired choice to the question was not included in the questionnaires (Rea & Parker 2005). Wording of the question should be clear to the subject. Avoid using words/sentence that can be interpreted in a variety of meanings or using abbreviations in the questions. It is because it may lead to difference in the interpretation between the respondent and the researcher and cause errors in the data collection. (McGibbon, 1997a).

The order of the questions should be put in logical way. Questions for similar items/categories should be grouped into a unit. It can be put into the following approach: chronologic, from general to specific, from easy to hard, from least sensitive to most sensitive, from most interesting and least interesting (Rattray & Jones, 2007). Appropriate spacing and font should be chosen to make the questionnaires look neat and tidy. It facilitates the respondent to read each question clearly and quickly. Put one single question per line. Title and clearly written instructions should be given at the beginning of the questions. If the questionnaires are more than one page, footnote "please continue at the next page" should be present to remind the respondent (Oppenheim, 1992). A statement to thank for the participation of respondent should be put at the end of the questionnaires. Small coding number for each category of the variables can be given at the side of the question to facilitate the data entry process afterward. Once the questionnaire has been developed, pilot test should be carried out on subjects who are similar to the desired respondents to test the validity and reliability of the questionnaire and discover the areas for improvement (Passmore, Dobbie, Parchman & Tysinger, 2002).

Questionnaires can be self-administrated, distributed by mail, e-mail or personally delivered. Since the researcher may not directly contact the subject, the researcher should follow some measures to facilitate the subjects to complete all the questions, e.g., short and attractive format and clear and concise invitation letter explaining the significance of this research to the subject (Sierles 2003). Researcher can provide some inducements to the subjects to enhance the response rate. It is not always in the form of money; it might be some convenience measure, e.g., self-addressed envelope (Fowler, 2009). The researcher should also be concerned about those people who did not respond to the survey. It is because this group may represent certain important missing parts and be passively "excluded" out of the research. The researcher should also try to find out the characteristics of these "missing" people, in order to be aware of any sampling bias or self-selection into the sample population and try to reduce such error (Choi & Pak, 2005).

As the characteristics of questionnaires mentioned above, we find that questionnaires can be used for obtaining information about feelings, values, opinions and motives from a large spectrum of subjects. Furthermore, a well-established questionnaire can provide a means for the participant to express their opinion directly. It can be appropriate for the application on the research about health issues or intervention in the large-scale nursing studies (Polit & Beck 2006).

# The Advantages and Disadvantages of the Observation Methods and Questionnaires

Both observational study and close-ended questionnaires are commonly used for assessing psychological and sociological variables in clinical settings. They can be applied to areas from investigating feeling, values, opinions to behavioral or attitude change after certain intervention. There are strengths and weaknesses to both methods.

There are a number of advantages to observation. Observation methods are a commonly used research tools, and they can be applied in a wide range of situations. The researcher can see directly the first-hand situation that is being studied. He/she can focus specially on the studying of the specific behaviors or activities. Moreover, the researcher can set the parameters of how much data they will collect. It relies less on the cooperation of a respondent. As a result, the researcher can achieve more control on the quality of data collection (Mateo & Kirchhoff, 1999.).

However, the major disadvantage of observation methods is its vulnerability to the bias of the observers. A person may impose or project his/her own distortions and biases unintentionally into his/her observation according to his/her own experience. Using multiple observers may help to reduce the level of individual bias. But meanwhile, it may lead to the differences of observations among the observers. Therefore, the researcher should train the observers carefully and provide appropriate guidelines or protocols to the observers to ensure the reliability of their observations in the study (Lobiondo-Wood et al. 2009). Another disadvantage of observation method is that the presence of an observer or camera during the observation process may cause the distortion of the subject's behaviors. It leads to the phenomenon called Hawthorne effect, in which the study subject tends to exhibit outcomes that they believe the researcher expects to see (Hulley et al., 2007). Observation method is also time consuming and labor intensive. The instruments for observers are often difficult and burdensome to construct and manage. Furthermore, there is also potential for violations of informed consent of privacy and confidentiality when people are observed (Caldwell & Atwal, 2005).

For the questionnaires, they are powerful data collection tools. They can obtain enormous amounts of information from large number of persons within a relatively short time. Uniformity of the responses in the questionnaires format also facilitates the data analysis. The standardized choices in the questionnaires facilitate the data analysis process. They can reduce the difference in the data perceptions among different researchers. A well-established questionnaire can be applicable for the similar research topics in different subject groups after the appropriate translation, validity and reliability tests. It is not necessary to create a new set of questionnaire every time when starting a new study with similar research focus. Furthermore, questionnaires also provide flexibility to the respondent by allowing the respondent to fill in and return the questionnaire during their free time (Fink, 2009).

Despite the above advantages, it is difficult and time consuming to generate a new questionnaire with significant validity and reliability when the researchers need to initiate research in a new area. It may take a lot of pretests and reviews during the construction process. Secondly, respondent bias is also a problem. Participant's answers are not reflective of true opinions. Sources of response bias reported by Topf (1986) include (1) carelessness (omit items, answer all items the same way, or do not follow the instruction), (2) social desirability, (3) acquiescence (tendency to agree), and (4) "central tendency" (consistently circling 3 when response choices range from 1-5). These biases can be reduced by 1) attaching a cover letter to explain the purpose of research and the significance of correct responses, 2) performing pretest to prove the clarity of instruction and items, 3) stating no right or wrong answers, 4) ensuring of confidentiality and 5) providing equal number of positive and negative choice responsively. Furthermore, as there may not be direct contact between the respondent and the researcher, people can refuse to join the study easily. Moreover, there may not be chance for the researcher and the respondent to verify the idea in the questionnaires. Misinterpretation may be aroused.

# Applications in Nursing Research

Observation methods and questionnaires can be applied in 1) answering the research questions in clinical setting (Knapp, 1998), 2) evaluating the effectiveness of nursing care (Santacroce, 2004; Whittemore, 2002), 3) expanding knowledge in nursing (Nieswiadomy, 2008). They are always used along with other research designs (e.g., experimental setting, intervention setting, biomedical instrumentation or interview) to increase the completeness and accuracy of the data collection and offset for the defect of different research methods, respectively (Brown, 2009). The following will use nursing researches in Hong Kong for discussion.

## Answering the Research Questions

During clinical practice, nurses always encounter questions about the nursing care or management of the ward. Nursing research provides a systematic process to find out the answers to those questions in clinical settings (Moule & Goodman, 2009). For example, Chang and Lam (1998) carried out a non-participant observation study on the role of healthcare assistants (HCA) and hospital-based training nursing students (SNs). In the late 1990s, the system of nursing education in Hong Kong changed from hospital-based to university-based. Hospitals service could no longer rely on the SNs. HCAs were introduced to assist qualified nurses to carry out patient care work. Questions arose that whether the introduction of HCA can replace the SNs? Would these changes leading to any difference in nursing role and manpower arrangement in the ward?

Chang and Lam divided the staff activities according to the working sampling component of the Patient Assessment and Information System (PAIS) into the following categories: 1) Direct patient care – including basic and technical nursing work; 2) Indirect activities – performed in the absence of the patients but did contribute to patient care; 3) Non productive activities – personal staff-related activities e.g., tea and meal breaks (Hovenga, 1990). The observational data was collected using Kruskal-Wallis' one-way analysis of variance. It was found that there were no significant differences in the total amount of all types of activities performed by SNs and HCAs. However HCAs were found to perform significantly less technical activities but more basic care than SNs. It implied that qualified staff may perceive that SNs had more knowledge and skills than HCAs and the SNs were assigned with more technical activities. It suggested that there was difference in the nature for the task assigned for the HCAs and SNs during the patient care process.

## Critique

Observation methods were applicable to study the staff activities in the ward setting in this study. However, the presence of a non-participant observer may lead to the distortion of the behavior of the staff. The instrument, the working sampling component of the PAIS, was clearly described. Validity and reliability of PAIS from previous study was reported but not for the current study. The number of observers and the training of observers were also not mentioned in this research paper.

## Implication

The introduction of HCA to replace the SNs probably causes changes in the nursing role e.g., 1) the nature and amount of the direct and indirect care activities carried out the qualified nurses; 2) difference in the ward management task of nurses e.g., changes in the amount of time and the strategies used for them to delegate and supervise unqualified staff.

## Evaluating the Effectiveness of Nursing Intervention

Nursing research can also be performed for evaluating the effectiveness of nursing interventions and patient care protocols (Polit & Beck, 2008). For example, Chan et al. (2007) used a self-administrated questionnaire to evaluate a community-based outreach breast health education program in pretest/posttest design from 2002 to 2003. Questions including the women's perceptions of health and disease of breast, perceptions of breast screening, practice and knowledge of breast self examinations (BSE), response if aware of any breast-related symptoms, willingness to pass this knowledge to friends and family, demographic data and breast cancer risk factor were included.

It was found that before the intervention, only 53.7 % of the participants were aware of breast health and breast diseases, and 48.6% were aware of breast screening methods. Women with more concern on the breast health and disease or had received instruction on BSE were more likely to have had experience in BSE practice before joining this program. However, after attending the health education program of breast health, most of the participants (77.7 to 93.7%) were capable to illustrate the method and timing for practicing BSE. Of the participants, 93.9% were willing to perform BSE regularly, and 92% of them were willing to share their knowledge on BSE with their relatives and friends. However, women with primary education or below tended to be insufficient in the knowledge about breast health and the effective utilization of the health care service when compared to the highly educated women.

## Critique and Implication

The comprehensiveness, validity and reliability of the instrument of this study was clearly described in this research paper. The use of pretest and posttest questionnaires in this study was an effective method to evaluate the validity of the health intervention in a large number of research subjects (777 people).

## Implication

The outreach health education program appeared to be useful for increasing the breast health awareness and BSE practice among the women. However, we suggested that there was a need for the healthcare professional to put more effort on the breast health promotion on the women with low education levels, as this group of women seemed not to be able to completely familiarize themselves with the use of the health care services.

## Expanding Nursing Knowledge

The nurses may get a lot of inspiration for research ideas throughout their clinical practice. On the other hand, researches generate knowledge to improve nursing practice. Conceptual frameworks and theories provide a structure of phenomena and are able to guide the direction study of clinical problems. They enable the focus of the inquiry by identifying the variables and concepts that are of interest and suggest the potential relationships among the variables and concepts. Conceptual frameworks and theories may possibly be proved when a relationship among variables is specified. Even if the theory or the specific relationships between or among variables and concepts were failed to be justified throughout testing, knowledge about the phenomenon is gained throughout the process. The testing of theories provides an important way for expanding knowledge (Houser, 2008).

For example, Kwong, Lam & Chan (2009) used Health Belief Model as a conceptual framework for the investigation of the factors that affect influenza vaccine uptake among community-dwelling Chinese elderly using the general outpatient clinics in Hong Kong. According to the modified Health Belief Model (Becker et al., 1977), the likelihood of an individual to perform a specific preventive behavior is affected by (1) how the he/she weighs the perceived benefits of and barriers to the preventive behavior; (2) how he/she perceives the threat of a specific illness, such as the susceptibility and severity of the illness, cues to actions and socio-demographic characteristics. The model had used to predict the individuals' influenza vaccination behavior (Armstrong et al., 2004) and other types of disease preventive behavior (Byrd, Peterson, Chavez & Heckert, 2004; Wai et al., 2005). The previous research found that the rate of receiving influenza vaccination in community-dwelling older Chinese people Hong Kong was low, 31.3% from 2003 to 2004 (Lau, Yang, Tsui & Kim., 2006). Therefore, Kwong, Lam & Chan carried out this study to investigate the factors affecting influenza vaccine uptake in this group of community-dwelling elderly. They recruited 197 subjects (aged 65 or above) from five Hospital Authority general outpatient clinics. A self-report questionnaire via face-to-face interview was used for data collection.

They found that 64.47% subjects reported having received the vaccine within the past 12 months. Factors influencing the elderly to receive vaccine were analyzed by the regression model. It revealed that those people with the health belief that "Vaccination prevents me from catching influenza," "If I get vaccinated, I will decrease the frequency of medical consultation" and "If I am vaccinated and still get flu, I will not be as sick with it," were more likely to receive the vaccination. On the contrary, people with the perception that "The side-effects of influenza vaccination interfere with my usual activities," "Influenza vaccination is painful," "I am scared of needles" prevent them from receiving vaccine. The recommendation from medical professionals and families also played a significant role in motivating the elderly to receive vaccination. It provides clues for the vaccination promotion strategies for the future.

## Critique

The research findings of this study were consistent with the conceptual model and the nature of the research question. The researcher adopted the self-report questionnaire for data collection via individual face-to-face interview, which can help to increase the response rate in the elderly subjects.

## Implication

As this group of elderly was more willing to accept the opinion from the medical professionals, nurses can take a role to encourage the community-dwelling elderly for receiving influenza by providing invitations, reminders and health talk of influenza vaccination specific for elderly. It is also important to include the family members of the elderly in the health education of influenza vaccination, as they may play an important role for enhancing the vaccinations received among the elderly.

# Conclusion

In this article, the characteristics, methodology, strengths, weaknesses and applications of observation methods and questionnaires in quantitative nursing research were discussed. Observation methods can be applied on the investigation of behavior and habit. It depends less on the cooperation of the subjects but it is time consuming and vulnerable to the bias of the observer. On the other hand, questionnaires can be applied on the investigation of attitude and opinion. It obtains information from the reflection of the subject. Questionnaires can be able to collect large amount of information with high uniformity in a relatively short period of time, but there is potential biases of self-report. Researcher can choose the research method according to the characteristics of variables and the purpose of their research.

# Author's Background

Tam Wing Yin is a Master of Nursing student in the Hong Kong Polytechnic University.

# References

Armstrong, K., Berlin, M., Schwartz, S., Propert, K., & Ubel, P. (2001). Barriers to influenza immunization in a low-income urban population. *American Journal of Preventive Medicine*, 20 (1), 21-25.

Becker, M. H., Haefner, D. P., Kasl, S. V., Kihscht, J. P., Maiman, L. A., & Rosenstock, I. M. (1977). Selected psychosocial models and correlates of individual health-related behaviours. *Medical Care*, 15 (Suppl.), 27–46

Brockopp, D. Y., & Hastings-Tolsma, M. T. (2003). *Fundamentals of Nursing Research*. Sudbury: Jones & Bartlett.

Brown, S. J. (2009). *Evidence-based Nursing: the Research-practice Connection*. Sudbury: Jones and Bartlett Publishers.

Burns, N., & Grove, S. K. (2007). *Understanding Nursing Research: Building an Evidence-based Pdractice*. Philadelphia: Elsevier Saunders.

Byrd, T. L., Peterson, S. K., Chavez, R., & Heckert A (2004). Cervical cancer screening beliefs among young Hispanic women. *Preventive Medicine*, 38 (2), 192–197

Casey, D. (2006). Choosing an appropriate method of data collection. *Nurse Researcher*, 13(3), 75–92.

Caldwell, K., & Atwal, A. (2005). Non-participant observation: using video tapes to collect data in nursing research. *Nurse Researcher*, 13(2), 42-54.

Chan, S. S., Chow, D. M, Loh, E .K., Wong, D. C., Cheng, K. K., Fung, W. Y., & Cheung, P. S. (2007). Using a community-based outreach program to improve breast health awareness among women in Hong Kong. *Public Health Nursing*, 24(3), 265-273.

Chang, A. M., & Lam, L. J. (1998). Can health care assistant replace student nurses? *Journal of Advanced Nursing,* 27 (2), 399-405.

Choi, B. C., & Pak, A. W. (2005). A catalog of biases in questionnaires. *Preventing Chronic Disease*, 2 (1), A13.

Dempsey, P. A., & Dempsey, A. D. (2000). *Using Nursing Research: Process, Critical Evaluation, and Utilization*. Philadelphia: Lippincott.

Fink, A. (2009). *How to Conduct Surveys: A Step by Step Guide*. Los Angels: SAGE.

Fowler, F. J. (2009). *Survey Research Methods*. Thousand Oaks: Sage Publications.

Gerish, K., & Lacey, A. (Eds.). (2006). *The Research Process in Nursing*. Oxford, UK; Malden, MA: Blackwell Publications.

Gillis, A., & Jackson, W. (2002). *Research for Nurses*: *Methods and Interpretation*. Philadelphia: F.A. Davis Co.

Houser, J. (2008). *Nursing Research: Reading, Using, and Creating Evidence.* Sudbury: Jones and Bartlett Publishers.

Hovenga, E. J. S. (1990). *The Origins of the Patient Assessment and Information System.* Melbourne: Health Department of Victoria, Melbourne, Australia.

Hulley, S. B., Cummings, S. R., Browner, W. S., Grady, D. G., & Newman, T. B. (2007). *Designing Clinical Research.* Philadelphia: Lippincott, Williams & Wilkins.

Jack, B. & Clarke, A. M. (1998). The purpose and use of questionnaires in research. *Professional Nurse*, 14(3), 176-179.

Knapp, T. R. (1998). *Quantitative Nursing Research.* Thousand Oaks: Sage Publications.

Kwong, E. W., Lam, I. O., & Chan, T. M. (2009). What factors affect influenza vaccine uptake among community-dwelling older Chinese people in Hong Kong general outpatient clinics? *Journal of Clinical Nursing*, 18 (7), 960-971.

Lau, J. T. F., Yang, X., Tsui, H. Y., and Kim, J. H. (2006). Prevalence of influenza vaccination and associated factors among community-dwelling Hong Kong residents aged 65 or above. *Vaccine*, 24 (26), 5526-5534.

Lobiondo-Wood, G., Haber, J., Cameron, C., & Sigh, M. D. (2009). *Nursing Research in Canada: Methods and Critical Appraisal for Evidence-based Practice.* Toronto: Mosby Elsevier.

Mateo, M. A., & Kirchhoff, K. T. (1999). *Using and Conducting Nursing Research in Clinical Setting* (2nd ed.). Philadelphia: W. B. Saunders Company.

Meadows, K. A. (2003). So you want to do research? Questionnaire Design. *British Journal of Community Nursing*, 8(12), 562-570.

McGibbon, G. (1997a). How to avoid the pitfalls of questionnaire design. *Nursing Times*, 93(19), 49-51.

McGibbon, G. (1997b). How to make a questionnaire work. *Nursing Times*, 93(23), 46-48.

Moule, P. & Goodman, M. (2009). *Nursing Research: An introduction.* Los Angles; London: SAGE.

Nieswiadomy, R. M. (2008). *Foundations of Nursing Research.* Upper Saddle River: Pearson/Prentice Hall.

Oppenheim, A. N. (1992). *Questionnaire Design, Interviewing and Attitude Measurement.* London; New York: Pinter Publishers.

Passmore, C., Dobbie, A. E., Parchman, M., & Tysinger J. (2002). Guidelines for constructing a survey. *Family Medicine*, 34(4), 281-286.

Polit, D. F., & Beck, C. T. (2006). *Essentials of Nursing Research: Methods, Appraisal, and Utilization*. Philadelphia: Lippincott Williams & Wilkins.

Polit, D. F., & Beck, C. T. (2008). *Nursing Research: Generating and Assessing Evidence for Nursing Practice*. Philadelphia: Wolters Kluwer Health/Lippincott Williams & Wilkins.

Rattray, J., & Jones, M. C. (2007). Essential elements of questionnaire design and development. *Journal of Clinical Nursing*, 16 (2), 234-243.

Rea, L. M., & Parker, R. A. (2005). *Designing and Conducting Survey Research: A Comprehensive Guide*. San Francisco: Jossey-Bass.

Santacroce, S. J., Maccarelli, L. M., & Grey, M. (2004). Intervention fidelity. *Nurisng Research*, 53 (1), 63-66.

Sierles, F. S. (2003). How to do research with self-administered surveys. *Academic Psychiatry*, 27 (2), 104-113.

Thom, B. (2007). Role of the simple, self-designed questionnaire in nursing research. *Journal of Pediatric Oncology Nursing*, 24 (6), 350-355.

Topf, M. (1986). Response sets in questionnaire research. *Nursing Research*, 35 (2), 119-121.

Wai, C. T., Wong, M.L., Ng, S., Cheok, A., Tan, M. H., Chua, W., Mak, B., Aung, M. O., & Lim, S.G. (2005). Utility of the health belief model in predicting compliance of screening in patients with chronic hepatitis B. *Alimentary Pharmacologic Therapy*. 21 (10), 1255–1262.

Whittemore, R., & Grey, M. (2002). The systematic development of nursing interventions. *Journal of Nursing Scholarships*, 34 (2), 115-120.

In: Clinical Research Issues in Nursing     ISBN: 978-1-61668-937-7
Editor: Z. C. Y. Chan, pp.119-128     © 2010 Nova Science Publishers, Inc.

*Chapter XI*

# Surveys for Clinical Research in Nursing

*Erin O. S. Cheng and*
*Zenobia C. Y. Chan*
The Hong Kong Polytechnic University, China

## Abstract

When we conduct research, we want to describe and explain a phenomenon. Sometimes, we can also predict a phenomenon and add knowledge onto the existing theory. The choice of research depends on the aim of the enquiry and the research questions to be answered. Quantitative research originates from positivism, and numerical data are collected. It is then analyzed by the statistical process under standard condition. Survey is one of the data collection methods commonly used in the clinical research. The survey design includes self-administered questionnaires, face-to-face interviews and interviews by telephone. This chapter will demonstrate a brief introduction of the research process, nature of the quantitative research, along with the survey designs. The advantages and disadvantages of using self-administered questionnaire and the situations of using the questionnaire for clinical research in nursing will also be reviewed.

# Literature Review on Research Paradigm

Clinical research is categorized according to its purpose and objectives (Masters et al., 2006), no matter which type of research, either quantitative, qualitative or mixed-mode research. The research process mainly includes research question identification, hypothesis establishment, research design selection, and data gathering, analyzing and interpreting so as to answer the research question (Kozier & Erb, 2008). One of the obvious distinctions between quantitative research and qualitative research is the research paradigm of data collection and the outcomes obtained. The outcomes obtained from the quantitative research can be measured using numerical data under standard conditions, while the measurement of qualitative research is obtained commonly from observing or interviewing the informants and in-depth meaning is gained (Endacott, 2008). This chapter aims to introduce one of the survey designs, self-administered questionnaire. Both the advantages and disadvantages of using questionnaires will be criticized so as to give a brief idea for the reader about the applications of questionnaire in different situations. Moreover, the situations of using surveys for clinical research in nursing will be illustrated.

# The Research Process

Clinical research is a systematic process with sequential steps in order to gain new knowledge or to verify the existing knowledge (Dempsey & Dempsey, 2000). The research process relies on empirical data or information collected. It allows a reasonable and logical framework for the study design. Hence, conclusion and generalization can finally be supported and derived from the verified data (Kozier & Erb, 2008; Portney & Watkins, 2009). The research process first starts with the identification of a research question for scientific testing that reveals the purpose of the study. It also controls the direction of all subsequent planning and analysis. Hypothesis is then established to clarify the research objective. Designing the study is a crucial step for planning the methods of subject selection, testing, and measurement. The measurements and interventions are defined to provide a clear method for data analysis (Whittier & George, 2009). Data collection is the implementation of the research plan, and it is the most time-consuming part in the research process. Enormous data are collected and a large database is developed, these raw data are reduced and analyzed into a useful form such as forms or tables. The remaining research process is data analysis, communication and sharing of findings with the appropriate audience (Portney & Watkins, 2009). The purpose of research is achieved because the information can be applied by others to clinical practice or to further research.

# Quantitative Research

Quantitative research is a systematic, scientific and logical strategy to collect information under the standard conditions of considerable control. It originates in positivism. It also assumes the reality is objective and can be measured or observed (Freshwater & Bishop, 2004; Crossan, 2003). Polit and Beck (2005) stated quantitative research was a philosophical doctrine that emphasized the rational and the scientific. It is often viewed as "hard" science, and it uses deductive reasoning with the measurable attributes of human experience. The most commonly used methods of collecting data in nursing are questionnaires, rating scales, interviews, observation, and biophysical measures. (Kozier & Erb, 2008)

In quantitative research, numeric data is usually collected under standardized conditions, and the data can be analyzed using conventional statistical methods (Peat, Mellis, Williams & Xuan, 2002). Quantitative information includes physical or physiological parameters such as the blood glucose level or the body mass index may be obtained. Moreover, the subjective information such as the pain level or degree of happiness is put into an objective numerical scale. It allows the researcher to summarize scales and subjective data to statistical analysis. The quantitative information is summarized into a meaningful way by the statistical procedures such as the SAS, SPSS, or STATA (Harwood & Hutchinson, 2009), and the decision of supporting or rejecting the research hypothesis will then be made (Portney & Watkins, 2009).

# The Applications of Survey

When types of data such as the subject characteristic or opinions are intended to be collected for the descriptive, exploratory or experimental studies, surveys or questionnaires are often used (Portney & Watkins, 2009).

Quantitative research often involves numerical data for which the sample size should be sufficiently large enough so that the data presented is deductive and representative of drawing the specific conclusion. Hence, a large database is developed and a secondary analysis is often used as a mechanism for exploring relationships. Surveys are widely and commonly used to collect information under two circumstances. They are when a large group of subjects are involved or when subjects need to define what level they agree on the situations given in a set of questions in a survey (Hek & Moule, 2006).

Surveys are good tools for obtaining information on a wide range of topics when in-depth probing of responses is not necessary, and they are useful for both formative and summative purposes. They are usually concerned with describing current practice, attitudes and values, characteristics of specific groups or identifying the general trends or patterns in data (Martin & Thompson, 2000). For instance, surveys are used at spaced intervals of time to measure the progress along some dimensions or changes in behavior. A series of questions posed to a group of subjects are included in a survey, and it may be conducted as an oral interview or as a written or electronic questionnaire. The data obtained from the surveys can vary in approaches and diversities that depend on the nature of the research design. The data can be targeted for the generalization to a larger population or as a description of a particular group. Despite the fact that both interviews and questionnaires are included in the categories of survey design, the discussion will focus on the applications of structured questionnaires only.

## Different Formats of Surveys

There are various formats of surveys; however, the basic components of the surveys always involve questions and responses. If the responses are intended to keep "open-ended," they allow the subjects to answer in a free flowing narrative form. However, the responses are most often kept as a "close-ended" approach, and the subjects are required to select from a range of predetermined answers adopted. There are benefits and difficulties with both "open-ended" and "close-ended" responses; the researchers have to make a decision on the applications of the particular responses. The decision is based on the nature of the research design and the appropriateness of the data collected or represented. Considering the "open-ended" responses, coding may be difficult and more time and resources may be required to handle than using the "close-ended" responses (Portney & Watkins, 2009; Gerrish & Lacey,

2006). A recommendation would be using a scale as a response because it facilitates the ease of the subjects to answer the questions, for instance, to give the agreement of the statement from 1 to 4 on a scale from "agree" to "disagree." Other than the degree of agreement measured on a scale, any different potential categories or issues that are difficult to be expressed in words and estimate such as period of time can also be measured and compared (Brockopp & Hastings-Tolsma, 2003).

There are many factors that would influence the distribution and collection of surveys including the complexity of questions, resources available and the project schedule. For instance, the data collection from the web-based surveys can be put directly into a database; the time and steps between data collection and analysis can be shortened. It also reduces the human resources in a research team that requires collecting and sorting the data manually. The responses are kept in the database with the computer-aided system, any out-of-range responses are possible to be checked and alerted. However, the web-based surveys require advanced technology and a significant resource to be invested. Hence, web-based surveys are appropriate to use when the surveys are fairly simple with no skip patterns and limited use of matrices.

# The Applications of Self-Administered Questionnaires

Questionnaire is a structured survey, and it is a self-administered form. It is designed to elicit data from the subject either through written or verbal responses (Gillis & Jackson, 2002). A self-administered form indicates the answers for the questionnaire provided by the subjects and can be given by pen and paper or electronic formats. It is more efficient because the subjects can complete the questionnaires whenever the time is convenient to them (Portney & Watkins, 2009). Under our considerations, giving out the questionnaires would be efficient to the researchers because a relatively short period of time is needed to gather the data from a large sample in a wide geographical distribution. Moreover, place is not necessary to be arranged if the questionnaires are available on the internet. It also allows the time for the subjects to think about their answers and to consult records for specific information. Another issue to be concerned with is the randomization of the sampling; if the sample is not large, it is necessary to promote the randomization. It ensures the probability of the results obtained is greater than pure chance (Knapp, 1998), and it can also avoid the bias of choosing a particular group. The questions in the questionnaire are standardized by the written forms, and all of the subjects are exposed to the same questions in the same way. The advantage of the standardization is to minimize the potential bias from interactions with an interviewer. No identity of the subjects such as their name, gender and contact are shown on the questionnaire, which provides anonymity, encouraging honest and candid responses. Furthermore, a questionnaire is particularly useful as a research method for examining phenomena that can be assessed through self-observation, for instance, attitudes and values (Portney & Watkins, 2009).

However, misunderstanding and misinterpreting the questions or response choices in the questionnaire from the subjects would be one of the major potentials to cause the false results (Portney & Watkins, 2009). It is also another problem for the subjects with reading difficulty or who are illiterate. It is also difficult to assess the accuracy and motivation of the subjects when they are answering the questionnaires. Unlike the interview, where the researchers have the chance to clarify the misinterpretations immediately, in a questionnaire, the researchers would only find the misinterpretation of subjects from the answers in the questionnaires during data analysis. It would be difficult to invite the same subjects to participate in the studies again, and it would obstruct the flow of the research. The most serious consequence is the lengthening of the research study. Hence, we recommend a short briefing on the questions, which can be provided to ease any misunderstanding of the questions. Moreover, questionnaires are not useful for studying behaviors that require objective observation.

## The Distributing Choice of Questionnaires

There are different methods of distributing questionnaires, for instance, through the mail, the electronic distribution, or in-person. The traditional distribution is through the mail or email, which takes time for delivering and receiving the questionnaires. The return rate of the questionnaires is low also. Responses from 60% to 80% of a sample are usually considered excellent. Realistically, researchers can expect return rates between 30% and 60% for most studies (Portney & Watkins, 2009). A recommendation would be a proper arrangement on returning the questionnaires. It can be achieved by discussing with the subjects to organize a convenient place and time for them to return the questionnaires. The researchers can also send email to the subjects if possible so as to remind them to complete and return the questionnaires. It improves the problem of low return rate. A large sampling size is important because it can minimize the effect caused by the limitation on the external validity of survey result.

In addition, actual response rates are lowered further by having to discard returns that are incomplete or incorrectly filled out. Low return rate can severely limit the external validity of survey result. In order to overcome the problem, survey samples are usually quite large so that a sufficient percentage of usable responses will be obtained. In contrast, if the questionnaires are distributed by the mean of electronic distribution, they allow anonymity and automatic tallying of responses. It is also economical and can reach a large population in a relatively short period.

The advantages and disadvantages of using surveys and questionnaires are summarized in Table 1.

## Table 1. The advantages disadvantages of using survey and questionnaires

| Advantages | Disadvantages |
|---|---|
| Information on a wide range of topics is obtained, but in-depth probing of responses is not necessary. Examples would be describing current practice, attitudes and values, characteristics of specific groups or identifying the general trends or patterns in data (Martin & Thompson, 2000). | The coding for "open-ended" responses may be difficult and more time and resources are consumed than using the "close-ended" responses (Portney & Watkins, 2009; Gerrish & Lacey, 2006). |
| Measuring in scale allows some issues which are difficult to be expressed in words and difficult to estimate such as period of time to be measured and compared (Brockopp & Hastings-Tolsma, 2003). | The traditional distribution of questionnaires through the mail or email which takes time for delivery and receiving. The return rate of the questionnaire is low also (Portney & Watkins, 2009). |
| It is more efficient for the subjects to complete the questionnaires whenever the time is convenient to them (Portney & Watkins, 2009). | Misunderstanding and misinterpreting the questions or response choices in the questionnaire from the subjects would be one of the major potentials to cause the false results (Portney & Watkins, 2009). |

# Surveys in Hong Kong

The data collection method of surveys and questionnaires has great implications for quantitative clinical research in Hong Kong, and it is commonly used in academic studies. One of the examples is a study conducted by Lau (2009) on the breastfeeding intention among pregnant Hong Kong Chinese women. A self-administered questionnaire is used to collect the demographic, socio-economic, and obstetric characteristics of the women. The findings suggest that effective promotion of breastfeeding during the prenatal period must target the correlates of feeding intention. Hence, as nurses, we can explain the benefits of breastfeeding and educate the method of breastfeeding to the pregnant women during their prenatal period. Another example is the study on women's knowledge about cervical cancer and cervical screening practice: a pilot study of Hong Kong Chinese women (Twinn, Shiu & Holroyd, 2002). In this case, quantitative and qualitative methods of data collection were both used, and they were the questionnaires and semistructured interviews, respectively. The study intended to investigate the level of knowledge about cervical cancer and cervical screening among Hong Kong Chinese women. The conclusion of this study demonstrated further knowledge about the preventive nature of cervical screening and regular screening were needed. Nurses can provide a culturally sensitive health promotion and implement the intervention strategies, such as encouraging women to have a regular screenings and seek medical help, if any signs and symptoms of cervical cancer are presented.

# Conclusion

As a conclusion, researchers have a responsibility to share their findings with the appropriate audience so that others can apply the information either to clinical practice or to further research. The purpose of data collection is to provide valid evidence to support the new knowledge gained from the research, and it improves our patient care.

# Author's Background

Erin O. S. Cheng is a Medical Laboratory Technician, and she is working in a private laboratory in Hong Kong. She is studying Master of Nursing currently. She wants to apply the knowledge learned from the Medical Laboratory Sciences into Nursing for better patient-centered care.

# References

Berman, A., Snyder, S. J., Kozier, B., & Erb, G. (2008). *Kozier & Erb's Fundamentals of nursing: Concepts, process, and practice.* (8th ed.). Upper Saddle River, N.J.: Pearson Prentice Hall.

Brockopp, D. Y., & Hastings-Tolsma, M. T. (2003). *Fundamentals of nursing research.* (3rd ed.). Boston: Jones and Bartlett.

Crossan, F. (2003). Research philosophy: towards an understanding. *Nurse Researcher.* 11(1), 46-55.

Dempsey, P. A., & Dempsey, A. D. (2000). *Using nursing research: Process, critical, evaluation, and utilization.* (5th ed.). Philadelphia, USA: Lippincott Williams & Wilkins.

Endacott, R. (2008). Clinical research 4: Qualitative data collection and analysis. *Journal of Emergency Nursing.* 16, 48-52.

Frechtling, J., Frierson, H., Hood, S., Hughes, G., & Katzenmeyer, C. (2002). *The 2002 User Friendly Handbook for Project Evaluation. Section III— An Overview of Quantitative and Qualitative Data Collection Methods.* The National Science Foundation. Retrieved December 4, 2009 from http://www.nsf.gov/pubs/2002/nsf02057/nsf02057_4.pdf.

Freshwater, D., & Bishop, V. (2004). *Nursing Research in Context: Appreciation, application and professional development.* Houndmills: Palgrave Macmillan.

Gerrish, K. & Lacey, A. (2006). *The research process in nursing* (5th ed.). Oxford: Blackwell Pub.

Gillis, A., & Jackson, W. (2002). *Research for Nurses: Methods and Interpretation.* Philadelphia: F.A. Davis Company.

Harwood, E. M., & Hutchinson, E. (2009). Data Collection Methods Series. Part 6: Managing Collected Data. *J Wound Ostomy Continence Nurs.* 36(6): 592-599.

Hek, G., & Moule, P. (2006). Making sense of research: *An introduction for health and social care practitioners.* (3$^{rd}$ ed.). London: Sage Publications Ltd.

Knapp, T. R. (1998). *Quantitative nursing research.* Thousand Oaks: Sage Publications, Inc.

Lau, Y. (2009). Breastfeeding Intention Among Pregnant Hong Kong Chinese Women. *Maternal and Child Health Journal.* 1-9.

Martin, C. R., & Thompson, D. R. (2000). *Design and Analysis of Clinical Nursing Research Studies: Routledge Essentials for Nurses.* London, N.Y; Routledge.

Masters, C., Carlson, D. S., & Pfadt, E. (2006). Winging it through research: an innovative approach to a basic understanding of research methodology. *Journal of Emergency Nursing.* 32(5), 382-384.

Muili, L. (2009). Reconciling methodological approaches of survey and focus group. *Nurse Researcher.* 17(1), 54-61.

Peat, J., Mellis, C., Williams, K., & Xuan, W. (2002). *Health science research: A handbook of quantitative methods.* London: Sage Publications Ltd.

Polit, D. F., & Beck, C. T. (2005). *Essentials of nursing research: Methods, appraisal, and utilization.* (6$^{th}$ ed.). Philadelphia: Lippincott Williams & Wilkins.

Polit, D. F., Beck, C. T., & Hungler, B. P. (2001). *Essentials of nursing research: Methods, appraisal, and utilization.* (5$^{th}$ ed.). Philadelphia, USA: Lippincott Williams & Wilkins.

Portney, L. G., & Watkins, M. P. (2009). *Foundations of clinical research application to practice.* Upper Saddle River, N.J.: Pearson Prentice Hall.

Twinn, S., Shiu, A. T. Y., & Holroyd, E. (2002). Women's knowledge about cervical cancer and cervical screening practice: a pilot study of Hong Kong Chinese women. *Cancer Nursing.* 25(5): 377-84

Whittier, S., & George, N. (2009). Research 101: Demystifying Nursing Research. *Home Healthcare Nurse,* 27(10), 635-639.

In: Clinical Research Issues in Nursing          ISBN: 978-1-61668-937-7
Editor: Z. C. Y. Chan, pp.129-139          © 2010 Nova Science Publishers, Inc.

*Chapter XII*

# Survey in Clinical Research

*M. Y. Siu and*
*Zenobia C. Y. Chan*
The Hong Kong Polytechnic University, China

There are ranges of data collection methods in quantitative research including interview, questionnaire, experiment, observation, etc. It is necessary for us to choose a suitable data collection method to suit the aims of clinical research. This chapter would concentrate on discussing the procedures, strengths, weaknesses and applications of survey: questionnaire and interview, because these are common and popular data collection methods (Saks & Allsop, 2007). Questionnaire is easy for beginners to follow because it does not need skillful interview and experimental knowledge when compared with the other data collection methods. However, researchers need to have well enough preparation to construct a set of validated and reliable questions for participants to "self-report" their opinions. Interview is administered by experienced interviewers to individuals for gathering additional information, opinions and points of view by face-to-face interaction with respondents. Through the whole interviewing process, interviewers are able to continuously evaluate the performance of respondents.

Survey design generally refers to sample survey (Vogt, 2007); sample is a group of individuals taken from a population (Wong, 2009) to make estimation about the population. It is used to collect quantitative data from large sample size by questionnaires and interviews. Survey is appropriate for descriptive and correctional studies (Hek & Moule, 2006). It is a logical thinking process by deductive approach that moves from the general conclusions to specific reasoning (Hek & Moule, 2006) to verify the existing knowledge and theory in order to achieve positivist approach of knowledge of quantitative research (Freshwater & Bishop, 2004). Objective, numeric and measurable data can be obtained by questionnaires and interviews. Quantitative researchers are interested in demonstrating a linkage and interrelationship between "cause and effect," e.g., the relationship of treatment and the outcome of the treatment. Survey is commonly used in quantitative research data collection method to explore causes, make predictions and study the relationships of various variables, which are classified as knowledge, attitudes, attribute, opinions and behaviors (Gillis & Winston, 2002).

This chapter has seven parts: a) closed-ended and open-ended questions; b) two types of survey questions; c) general guidelines for administering survey questions; d) procedures of constructing survey design; e) strengths and weaknesses of questionnaires and interviews; f) discussion and g) conclusion.

# Closed-ended and Open-ended Questions

For quantitative research, closed-ended questions have higher proportion than open-ended questions because closed-end questions are more suitable for data analysis.

# Closed-ended Questions

The following content was abstract from Burnard & Morrison (1994). The wording of closed-ended questions are predetermined as structured-typed questions with a number of fixed alternatives for respondents to choose, including dichotomous, multiple choice, cafeteria, ranking order, forced choice, rating, checklist (Polit & Beck, 2010), which are questions easy for respondents to choose from. This is done to ensure the consistency in the range of answers. It is easy for respondents to handle and for us to analyze data, for example: "Does the patient turn his head while feeding?" (Watson, 1996)

Questionnaire is an effective method because respondents are able to complete more closed-ended questions than open-ended question in a given amount of time. However, it is challenging to construct a set of validated and reliable questions. Clinical researchers have to improve and modify the questions for respondents to make them easy to understand, in order to get the necessary information to achieve purposes and aims of the clinical research project.

# Open-ended Questions

The below content was referenced from Burnard & Morrison (1994). Open-ended questions are unstructured-type questions that often begin with what, why, where, when and how. Respondents use their own words to answer the open-ended questions. Questions are asked for respondents to write down the opinions by clinical researchers and opinions to get the additional information as a light to make recommendations and new issues have been arisen for future clinical researches. It can be used to measure the beliefs, attitudes, opinions and knowledge of participants.

# Two Types of Survey Questions

There are two major types of survey questions: attitude questions and behavioral questions. Attitudinal questions consist of a series of questions regarding the feeling, behaviors, experience, point of view (Burnard & Morrison, 1994), even evaluation and judgment (Sudman, Bradburn & Schwarz, 1996) of respondents about a situation. Behavioral questions are information and memory, such as the type of activity, time, venue and attendants of events that provide important information to linking cause and effect relationship (Sudman, Bradburn & Schwarz, 1996).

# General Guidelines for Administering Survey Questions

| Rule 1: Establish Legitimacy |
| --- |
| Consent of participants must be collected. At the beginning of survey, the length of time of interview or questionnaire, times of data collection and the importance and purpose of the survey to the society and health care system of the clinical research should be clearly stated to eliminate misunderstanding. The professional wordings can build up confidence of subjects, and researchers must guarantee their answer confidentiality and anonymity (Vogt, 2007). |
| Rule 2: Easy for subjects to understand |
| The questions must be easy for participants to understand to prevent misinterpretation (Gillis & Winston, 2002). |
| Rule 3: Relevancy of questions |
| The questions must be relevant to the research topics and cover various scopes to enrich the information (Moule & Goodman, 2009). |
| Rule 4: Respect to participants |
| Do not force subjects to join the study (Gillis & Winston, 2002). Must respect people who do not wish to take part in the study because the study may conflict their personal beliefs and values. And respect the right of subjects throughout the whole processes during collecting data (Chan, 2009). |
| Rule 5: Quality control |
| The study should administrate and monitor the regulated procedures to maintain the validation and reliability of the study (Gillis & Winston, 2002) by careful planning and management (Saks & Allsop, 2007). |

# Procedures of Constructing Survey Design

In fact, the procedures of collecting data by questionnaire and interview are similar. There are few differences between them.

The following procedures were adopted from Bruce & Pope (2008), Burnard & Morrison (1994), and Gillis & Winston (2002).

Literature review and construction of the instrument, e.g., questionnaire, are the most time-consuming parts of quantitative research. We should have deep investigation about the past nursing research in order to determine the significance of our current research.

| |
|---|
| Formulate research question to guide the study (Knapp, 1998) and define the aims, objectives, hypothesis and targets of the clinical research. |
| Select the type of survey that should be used in the study, e.g., questionnaires, face-to-face interview or phone interview. |
| Collect necessary information and define requirement that are needed to achieve and fulfill the targets. |
| Literature reviews: take reference of related topics that are prior to this study to get new information and argument from other scholars to enrich our knowledge, analyze the current existing problems of the clinical research topic from clinical experience, nursing literature, social issues and theories (Polit, Beck, & Hungler, 2001). |
| Translate the objectives of survey into categories of questions and define the type of questions: Closed-ended questions that are easy for subjects to answer the questions in given amount of time. Open-ended questions to take the additional information from respondents. |
| Determine the sample size, response rate and selection of sample from population: probability to increase generalization and applications of clinical research. |
| Consider what kinds of relevant information and opinions should be asked by clinical researchers with the consideration of cultural and environmental factors. |
| Adopt and modify the existing and tested instruments that meet our requirements or build up a set or draft new questions by our innovation to be relevant to the objectives and free of bias. |
| Design data collection procedures and plan for data analysis. |
| At the beginning, the length and purpose of the questionnaire and interview should be clearly stated to the targeted subjects (Moule & Goodman, 2009). Promise to keep confidentiality and anonymity of their responsive answers (Vogt, 2007). |
| Pre-test / Pilot test: the approaches for data collection and data analysis to write down the existing problems of a series of set of questions (Bruce & Pope, 2008) and identify solution to overcome the factors that may affect the conduction of the study, including the availability, work load and restriction to assess the participants (Chan, 2009). |
| Modify the exiting series of set questions and procedures as necessary to suit the current situation, then questionnaire is ready to use. |
| Distribute the questionnaire / make an appointment with the respondents to arrange interview schedule of face-to-face interviews or phone interview when they are available of their own free will and feeling comfortable in the interviewing environment to complete the questions. |
| Pay attention to the feedback of respondents. |
| Collect data from participants and keep information confidential. |
| Analyze data by using suitable statistical skills. Draw conclusions to finalize the study. |

# Strengths and Weaknesses of Questionnaires and Interviews

Questionnaires and interviews each have their advantages and disadvantages; it depends on type of information that clinical researchers need.

# Questionnaires

Questionnaires are effective data collection methods that mainly depend on closed-ended questions to save time and to make it easy for data analysis.

## Strengths and Weaknesses of Questionnaire

| Strengths | Weaknesses |
|---|---|
| Effective and save time to collect much data from a large number of subjects (Burnard & Morrison, 1994). | There are no direct interactions between the respondents and clinical researchers. Clinical researchers may overlook some potential important responses of clinical researches through self-report type questions (Burnard & Morrison, 1994). |
| Cost effective method: Less money will be spent, it is suitable for clinical research that has limited amount of clinical research fund (Burnard & Morrison, 1994). | Construction of a validated and reliable questionnaire is not an easy task (Burnard & Morrison, 1994). |
| Questionnaire can be completed in group settings or disturbed through internet and mail even though the samples are geographically dispersed all over the world (Polit & Beck, 2010). | The questions may be misinterpreted and misunderstood by the respondents (Moule & Goodman, 2009). |
| Eliminate interviewers' bias: The responses of respondents are not disturbed by the clinical researchers and the other respondents, because questionnaire is mainly self administered (Polit & Beck, 2010). | The response rate and feedback is low (Moule & Goodman, 2009). |
| Support anonymity: Questionnaire can provide enough privacy to respondents. The respondents would tell the facts to the clinical researchers even though when they are answering sensitive and embarrassing questions, the accuracy of answers is high (Polit & Beck, 2010). | Questionnaires rely on closed-ended questions (Bruce & Pope, 2008), so the choice of responses has been set by the interviews, e.g., dichotomous, checklist, multiple choices & rank order, etc. (Burnard & Morrison, 1994). |

| Strengths | Weaknesses |
| --- | --- |
| Self completion: Participants can complete the questionnaires when they are available and convenient. | Return of incomplete questionnaires, however, it may not be possible to go back to the respondents (Bruce & Pope, 2008). |
| Engage large amount of samples in a given period of time even though when there are human resources limitation between clinical researchers and participants, so it is extremely suitable for small clinical research team to overcome power issues with limited data collection time (Moule & Goodman, 2009). | Questionnaires are not suitable to group of people (Wong, 2009), for example, blind people, illiterate people, individuals with mental illnesses, young children, very ill and elderly. |
| The type of questions can be set according to the data analysis method of the clinical research design with respect to suitable statistical technique (Moule & Goodman, 2009). | No additional opinions, feelings and emotions of respondents can be experienced by the interviewers. |
| No need to perform the clinical research with well-prepared equipment. | The language of questionnaires must be understandable by the participants. |
|  | The questionnaire must not be long or complex (Bruce & Pope, 2008). |

# Interviews

Although questionnaire is an effective method, there are various limitations. However, the strengths of interviews outweigh the limitations of questionnaires. There are requirements of interviewers to collect data without adding personal, self-centered values and subjective opinions to participants. Observations can be gathered through face-to-face interviews.

There are different types of interviews: face-to-face interviews, telephone interviews and group interviews (focus group interviews).

# Strengths and Weaknesses
# of Interviews

| Strengths | Weaknesses |
| --- | --- |
| The response rate is high, with less refusal rate: Good rapport has been established through the interaction of interviews between interviewers and participants. Participants are willing to answer the questions of interviewers to keep high response rate (Gillis & Winston, 2002). | Interview is time consuming and costly procedure (Bruce & Pope, 2008). |

**(Continued).**

| Strengths | Weaknesses |
|---|---|
| When respondents have some questions regarding the interview questions, chances have been provided for interviewers to give clarification and explanation to ensure participants understand all the questions and prevent misinterpretation of respondents (Bruce & Pope, 2008). | Limited generalization: The sample size of interview would be much lower than questionnaire (Saks & Allsop, 2007). |
| Interviewer can observe the facial expression, reluctance, living environment, etc., of participants when they are expressing the experiences and opinions. | Interviewers' bias: the distortion of response due to the performance and interviewing skill of interviewers would have great impact on the quality of collected data. (Bruce & Pope, 2008; Gillis & Winston, 2002). The interviewers must be humble, objective, respective and not self centered. They need to take the role as aside and take the balance between participants and observers. |
| Interviewers are able to continue evaluating, adjust the questions, draw additional attention to important issues and explore issues more open ended questions in more depth (Bruce & Pope, 2008) with respect to response and culture of respondents though the process of interview. | If the research is carried out by more than one interviewer, standardized training should be provided for interviewers to ensure the accuracy and credibility of data result (Bruce & Pope, 2008). |
| There is time for interviewers to edit the existing question set and redefine the clinical research directions before the beginning of next interview. | Retention of subjects: when respondents are answering sensitive questions, they may adjust and alter the answer accordingly to fit the situation. |
|  | Slow recruitment and the availability of respondents would lengthen the clinical research time for collection data. |

# Discussion

   Survey is probably an extremely popular used data collection method in practice of local clinical researches for students and scholars to obtain objective information from a selected population (hospitals and the public). Journal publication is the most common medium to share result of studies (Mateo & Kirchhoff, 1991). The subjects of clinical researchers are the health care providers (the nurse and doctors), for example, nurses' perception of disaster (Fung , Lai, & Loke, 2009) and the health care receivers (the patients and family members). The type of questions can be adjusted according to the objectives of the clinical researches and in addition to knowledge and cultural background of participants. It can be used to collect large number of information from the sampling data for evaluating the level of public satisfaction with local health care, improving the existing Hong Kong health care system, getting opinions of subjects to evaluate the room for upgrading the standard of care and service provided for the clients in Hong Kong. In recent years, scholars have used survey as data collection method to conduct quantitative research, such as investigating the relationship of contraceptive self-efficacy and contraceptive knowledge with unplanned pregnancy of Chinese Hong Kong women (Ip, Sin, & Chan, 2009); the importance of social support and coping effectiveness of Chinese patients undergoing cancer surgery (Chan, Hon, Chien, & Lopez, 2004); the importance of educational needs of families caring for Chinese patients with schizophrenia (Chien & Norman, 2003).

Longitudinal and cross-sectional study should be taken into consideration before the beginning of study. Longitudinal study is able to measure changes over time. During different points of time and time series, trends are monitored over time, the views and opinions of respondents would be altered before and after treatment, the outcome of the result will be changed accordingly.

Surveys are major tools in local clinical researches to represent large population by selecting appropriate sampling and suitable sample size. However, there are common limitations of survey that are beyond the control of researchers when collecting information. There are slow recruitment rate of subjects with regard to the availability and current work load of participants, insufficient potential subjects (Chan, 2009) to meet the generalization, clinical researchers who are not able to approach and invite potential subjects to join the study. It is important to determine the response rate in survey. There are certain retentions of the participants to interrupt the data result.

# Conclusion

Data collection is a challenging part of a clinical research study of the Hong Kong health field. Clinical researchers have to consider the response of subjects, accuracy of data collected and the response rate of respondents, time series of collecting data and the background information of respondents by sample selection to ensure the validity and reliability of study.

Questionnaire and interview have their potential strengths and weaknesses. The combination of both data collections can enrich the information of collected data and outweigh their limitations, in order to construct a validated and reliable clinical research study. Methodological triangulation with mixed methodology design (Freshwater & Bishop, 2004) is a solution to outweigh the weakness of different methods. However, it is time consuming and increases the difficulties in data analysis (Chan, 2009). Clinical researchers need to have good time management to integrate different methods in a single study.

# References

Bruce, N. & Pope, D. (2008). *Quantitative methods for health research: a practical interactive guide to epidemiology and statistics,* Chichester ; Hoboken, N.J.: John Wiley & Sons.

Burnard, P. & Morrison, P. (1994). *Nursing research in action: developing basic skills (2nd ed.).* Basingstoke, Hampshire: Macmillan Press.

Chan, C. W., Hon, H. C., Chien, W. T., & Lopez, V. (2004). Social support and coping in Chinese patients undergoing cancer surgery. *Cancer Nursing, 27*(3), 230-236.

Chan, C. Y. (2009). *Lecture notes of Clinical Research Studies.* Hong Kong: The Hong Kong Polytechnic University.

Chien, W. T., & Norman, I. (2003). Educational needs of families caring for Chinese patients with schizophrenia. *Journal of Advanced Nursing, 44*(5), 490-498.

Freshwater, D. & Bishop, V. (2004). *Nursing research in context: appreciation, application and professional development.* Basingstoke: Palgrave Macmillan.

Fung, W. M., Lai, K. Y., & Loke, A. Y. (2009). Nurses' perception of disaster: Implications for disaster nursing curriculum. *Journal of Clinical Nursing, 18*(22), 3165-3171.

Gillis, A. & Winston, J. (2002). *Research for nurses: methods and interpretation.* Philadelphia, Pa.: F.A. Davis Co.

Hek, G. & Moule, P. (2006). *Making sense of research: an introduction for health and social care practitioners (3rd ed.).* London: Sage Publications Ltd.

Ip, W. M., Sin, L. Y. & Chan, S. K. (2009). Contraceptive self-efficacy and contraceptive knowledge of Hong Kong Chinese women with unplanned pregnancy. *Journal of Clinical Nursing, 18* (17), 2416-2425.

Knapp, T. R. (1998). *Quantitative nursing research.* Thousand Oaks, Calif.: Sage Publications.

Mateo, M. A. & Kirchhoff., K. T. (1991). *Using and conducting nursing research in the clinical setting (2nd ed.).* Philadelphia: W.B. Saunders.

Moule, P. & Goodman, M. (2009). *Nursing research: an introduction.* London: Sage Publications Ltd.

Polit, D. F., Beck, C. T. & Hungler., B. P. (2001). *Essentials of nursing research: methods, appraisal & utilization (5th ed.).* Philadelphia: Lippincott.

Polit, D. F. & Beck, C. T. (2010). *Essentials of nursing research: appraising evidence for nursing practice (7th ed.).* Philadelphia, PA: Wolters Kluwer Health/Lippincott Williams & Wilkins.

Saks, M. & Allsop, J. (2007). *Researching health: qualitative, quantitative and mixed methods.* London: Sage Publications Ltd.

Sudman, S., Bradburn, N. M. & Schwarz, N. (1996). *Thinking about answers: the application of cognitive processes to survey methodology (1st ed.).* San Francisco: Jossey-Bass Publishers.

Vogt, W. P. (2007). *Quantitative research methods for professionals.* Boston, Mass.: Pearson/Allyn and Bacon.

Watson, R. (1996). The mokken scaling procedure (MSP) applied to the measurement of feeding difficulty in elderly people with dementia. *International Journal of Nursing Studies, 33*(4), 385-393.

Wong, A. (2009). *Lecture notes of Clinical Research Studies: Quantitative research method.* Hong Kong: The Hong Kong Polytechnic University.

In: Clinical Research Issues in Nursing                    ISBN: 978-1-61668-937-7
Editor: Z. C. Y. Chan, pp.141-150            © 2010 Nova Science Publishers, Inc.

*Chapter XIII*

# Ethics in Nursing Research

## *F. H. Tang[1,] and*
## *Zenobia C.Y. Chan[1]*
[1] The Hong Kong Polytechnic University, China

## Abstract

Ethics is a sense of right and wrong morally. Ethics applied in clinical research stated what ought and ought not to be done in a research. It ensures the quality of research and protects the rights of human subjects. There are different principles and theories in ethics, and it is important to take a balance in between. Although different guidelines and research ethics committees exist in different countries, the core elements of the ethics are universal. Researchers should strictly follow the guidelines and get approval before the conducting a research. A good ethical consideration should take a balance on the safety, the scientific needs and the ethical acceptability. Virtue and integrity must be upheld during the research.

## Introduction

Ethics is a sense of being right or wrong of an action morally. It might contradict the code of practice and lead to ethical dilemmas. Hence, ethics is often applied for criticizing and promoting moral concepts in our daily practice (Newall, 2005). Ethics being applied in the clinical research emphasizes what ought and ought not to be done in a research involving human subjects. It emphasizes the value of conducting a research and protects the right of subjects (Moss, 2005, p.3-4). This essay aims to study the schools of ethics and the importance of ethics in clinical research. Books, journals and different guidelines of ethics were gone through to gather the existing information about ethics. The focus and the weakness of schools of ethics are discussed with support from the existing information. However, it is just a brief study of ethics; hence many areas can be further exposed.

In the following, a brief history of the introduction of ethics is reviewed; the types of ethics and its importance are examined; elements and the strategy to ensure ethics are studied; and finally, the ethics system of clinical research in Hong Kong is examined.

# History of the Code of Ethics

The introduction of code of ethics was highlighted after the Second World War (Tadd, 2003). During the Second World War, large amounts of biomedical experiment researches were held. These researches were conducted without the acknowledgement of participants and caused irreversible damage to their health, such as Tuskegee syphilis study and Willowbrook study. In Tuskegee syphilis study, blacks were exposed to syphilis without acknowledgement and further treatment after the research, which resulted in a life-long disease suffered by the participants (Tadd, 2003). In Willowbrook study, mentally handicapped children were exposed to hepatitis virus involuntarily (Tadd, 2003). These inhuman activities alerted the public concern on the ethical issue, and hence the first code of ethics, called Nuremberg Code, was created in 1948. It aims to restrict the researches on human subjects by setting out standards to measure the rights of the participants (Dempsey & Dempsey, 2000; Dempsey & Goodman, 2009). It was then modified and named the declaration of Helsinki in 1964, which is a protocol of many later regulations (Dempsey & Dempsey, 2000).

# Ethical Principles and Guidelines

## Belmont Report

There are different principles of ethics. The most common principle to be considered is Belmont Report. It acts as a guide to verdict the ethical stipulation and researches, which involves human subjects.

## Respect for Persons

Respect for persons states that the self-determination and full disclosure of participants should be respected. For those with insufficient autonomy, their autonomy should be protected by an authorized surrogate (Ruan, Brady & Cooke, 1979; Portney & Watkins, 2009; Adam, 1999).

## Beneficence

Beneficence emphasizes that research conduction should maximize the possible goods and minimize the possible harm in a research (Adam, 1999; Moss, 2005; Ruan, Brady & Cooke, 1979).

## Justice

Justice indicates that research should be conducted in a fair distribution. Benefits and the burdens should be equally distributed according to the participant's needs, their efforts and contribution to the society (Ruan, Brady & Cooke, 1979; Portney, 2009; Adam, 1999).

Belmont Report provides a general principle of ethics to be followed during the research with human involvement. It enhances researchers' concern on the rights of the patients. However, these principles are too general and lack specific judgment; therefore it cannot ensure the quality of ethics to be upheld (Moss, 2005). A more specific guideline is required to justify and maintain a good quality ethics in clinical research.

In order to analyzes how to maintain the ethics principle within the research, theories of ethics were introduced, which include consequentiality ethical theory, deontology and virtue ethics

## Consequentiality Ethical Theory

Consequentiality ethical theory focused on the outcome. According to the theory, the meritorious of actions is directly proportional to the goods for the majority. It allows researches to place subjects into little harm if an important message or knowledge can be obtained (Moss, 2005).

This theory encourages researchers to put the beneficence of future patients and society on the highest priority. It is an important theory applied in the research as every research contains potential risk due to the uncertainty of outcome (Moss, 2005). However, if the theory is applied immoderately, it may override the principle of ethics and cause irreversible damage to participants or even death. As a result, a well-equilibrium balance of risks and benefits should be achieved before researches.

## Deontology

Deontology emphasizes the obligation or duties of the clinical researchers and the willingness of subjects. The input to the research and the right of the participants are treated far more importantly than the outcome (Kay, 1997).

Participants are the main concern in the theory that researchers should be responsible for them. Furthermore, their dignity and autonomy of the patient should be maintained. To do so, informed consent with full descriptions of the research is essential to protect the right of participants. Besides, additional body for investigation is necessary to reduce the blind point of protecting human subjects in the research (Moss, 2005).

## Virtue Ethics

Virtue ethics focused on the virtue of the researcher. It states that researchers should never put the subject at a risk of unacceptable harm, no matter how beneficial the research is (Moss, 2005).

This theory put a highlight on the protection of participants from the risk of harm. However, it might be difficult to apply in real practice, as all researches are carrying some unknown issues, which may do harm to the subject. Instead, applying this theory to the clinical research, we should minimize the harm to the subjects.

To summarize, there is no definite answer for which theory should be more emphasized or applied. Different theories have their own strengths and weaknesses. Researchers should take a balance in theories and avoid going to either extreme. A good ethical consideration should take a balance on the safety, the scientific needs and the ethical acceptability. Virtue and integrity must be upheld in the research.

# Importance of the Ethics

Ethics is a significant part, which must be continuously considered in researches. It examines the value of the research by taking an equilibrium on the benefits from the research and the potential harm to subjects. It protects the rights of participants with autonomy, freedom of participation and consideration of risk-benefits ratio. It is a core element to be considered in a research. In many cases, development of a new knowledge may lead to unpreventable harm to subjects due to the error of estimation and uncertainties. Timely review of the procedure and the risk-benefits ratio is required to examine the value of the continuity of study. Sometimes, researches may be valid, but there may lead to unacceptable damage to participants, like those experiments in the Second World War. Ethics plays an important role by putting an eye on the protection of subjects to prevent unnecessary or unacceptable damages by stating what must and must not be conducted. Moreover, it ensures the quality of the research and services provided and hence, enhances the public confidence in clinical research.

# Elements to Be Considered

Ethics is not a single issue to be considered. It may be affected by different components in the research. Five major elements to be considered were stated by the Research governance framework as shown below (Moule & Goodman, 2009).

## Science

Research should build on top of existing knowledge. A thorough literature review is essential before the research to gather the existing knowledge. Knowledge gap should be identified before the conduction of research to ensure the value of conducting a research. Besides, it should be conducted by qualified researcher to ensure the quality and the safety (Moule & Goodman, 2009). Proposals should be explored by peers for advice and submitted to the legal committee to ensure meeting the good ethical standard and identify potential risks (Moule & Goodman, 2009). Validity of the data should be examined, as it may directly influence the quality and the value of the research.

## Information

The information should be well organized and accessible. Data should be controlled in confidential manner to protect the privacy of subjects such that no identifying data will be exposed to the public. There are a couple of ways to ensure the confidentiality, which include getting confidential assurance among the research group members, securing identifying data by a locking system with access control, assigning a number for identification rather than the personal information (Polit & Beck, 2008).

## Health and Safety

Safety should be placed on top of any other issues in the research. Risk should be identified before the data collection. A risk-benefit assessment should be done regularly to ensure that the risk of harm is minimized and never exceed the potential benefits. Debriefings and referrals may be required after the data collection to provide support and clear up the queries or harm associated with the research (Polit & Beck, 2008).

## Finance and Intellectual Property Ethics

Researchers should have a clean hand from the public funding and the usage in intellectual property, which should be monitored legally. Proper reference is important to prevent plagiarism Besides,, the relationship between funders and the research should be reviewed before accepting any funding to ensure the design and the implementation will not be influenced (Bass, Dunn & Norton, et al., 1993; Moule & Goodman, 2009).

## Ethics

The dignity, safety and the right of participants are significantly important. An informed consent with a witness is necessary to protect the rights of participants. The nature of studies and the possible harm and goods should be fully informed before making the decision of participation. The quality of service should not be influenced with the decision. Confidentiality and autonomy should be protected with the security of data storage. Proposal should be sent to the independent ethics committee for approval to ensure the good ethical standard. Risk should be minimized before the conduction of research and should be examined continuously (Moule & Goodman, 2009). Researches should be completed unless they are causing unacceptable harm because giving up a research might cut off the benefits to the future patients, which is also unethical.

Ethics is not an individual component to be considered. Poor scientific approach may affect the quality of ethics. The five dimensions have stated the main components and interventions to be carried out in order to optimize a good quality research. Ethical consideration should be raised early in the planning stages and keen on the rest of the research. Apart from this, external review in each element may be required to strengthen the quality of ethics by providing different stand points and pointing out blind points in the research.

# Ethics Committee in Hong Kong

Different countries do have their own ethics committee to monitor their ethical standard of researches. They are empowered by law and respected by the authority. Although there may be small variation between their guidelines due to the differences in the cultures and the judicial traditions, the core elements of ethics are synchronized (Tadd, 2003). In Hong Kong, there is no specific statute focusing on the clinical research (Hospital Authority, 2008). Instead, there is Code of Professional Conduct, which was developed by the Medical Council of Hong Kong as a guideline for all clinical researches.

Besides, Research Ethics Committees (REC) is established by the Hospital Authority to review and monitor the studies.

REC is made up by the HAHO Steering Committee on Research Ethics and the Cluster REC. Cluster REC is responsible for the approval of research proposals and any changes such that no research should be conducted before the ratified of the committee. It also monitors the progress of the research and has the authority to pause the suspected studies, which may be harmful to subjects. HAHO Steering Committee on Research Ethics is responsible for establishing guidelines for ethics and risk management. These guidelines are equivalent to the international standard, in addition to handling appeals against the judgment of Cluster REC (Hospital Authority, 2007).

Apart from monitoring the research progress, REC also provides education on the research conduct and ethical review through the internet and training courses. For example, The University of Hong Kong, as the partners of the Hong Kong West Cluster REC, together with Queen Mary Hospital has developed a platform called ClinCluster, which provides support in different phases of research (ClinCluster, 2004).

REC is playing an important role in the contribution of good ethical standard in Hong Kong. It enhances the quality of ethics by monitoring the researches and educating researchers. The supportive service of the REC takes a significant role in facilitating the practice. However, there is no strict regulation specific to the clinical research in Hong Kong. As a result, self-discipline of the research group is taking a more important role in this aspect.

# Conclusion

To conclude, ethics is a significant issue to be considered continuously. It aims to state what should and should not be done in a research. It protects the rights of human subjects and ensures the quality of research. Under the consideration of ethics, we should not give up a study unless it will lead to unacceptable harm, as giving up will terminate the potential benefits of the study to the society. A good quality of ethics consideration should take a balance on the safety, the scientific needs and the ethical acceptability. Virtue and integrity must be upheld during the research. To ensure the quality of ethics, there are several international guidelines. Although there may be variations due to the differences in culture and policy, the core elements are universal. Reviewing the ethics conducting system in Hong Kong, although there is no legal regulation, well-established guidelines and committees are available. Support is given to facilitate the understanding and assist in the application for the good clinical practice. This has resulted in a good ethical clinical research practice in Hong Kong. However, the existing regulation system is under the Hospital Authority. This may influence the education and policy of the ethics committee to be Hospital Authority-oriented. Hence, an independent research ethics committee is needed for further improvement to target professional from all aspects.

# References

Adam, R. N. (1999). Ethics and nursing research 1: development, theories and principles. *British Jouranl of Nursing, 8*(13), 888-892.

Bass, M. J., Dunn, E. V., Notron, P. G., Wtewart, M. & Tudiver, F. (1993). *Conducting research in the practice setting.* Newbury Park: Sage Publications.

ClinCluster Portal: The Gateway to ClinCluster (2004). Retrieved November 3, 2009 from ClinCluster, Web site: http://www.clincluster.com/ser.html.

Dempsey, P. A., & Dempsey, A. D., (2000). *Using nursing research: process, critical evaluation, and utilization, 5th Edition.* Philadelphia: Lippincott.

Handbook for Good Clinical Research Pracitce: Gudiance for Implementation (2002). Retrieved December 4, 2009 from World Health Origanization, Web site: http://ori.dhhs.gov/documents/WHOHandbookonGCP04-06.pdf.

Hospital Authority (HA) Clinical Research Study Site Guide (2004). Retrieved October 10, 2009 from Hospital Authority, Research Ethics Committee Web site: http://www.ha.org.hk/ho/research_ethics/hare002.pdf.

Hospital Authority (HA) Guide on Research Ethics (2007). Retrieved October 10, 2009 from Hospital Authority, Research Ethics Committee Web site: http://www.ha.org.hk/ho/research_ethics/hare004.pdf.

Hospital Authority (HA) Investigator's Code of Practice(2004). Retrieved October 10, 2009 from Hospital Authority, Research Ethics Committee Web site: http://www.ha.org.hk/ho/research_ethics/hare003.pdf.

Research Ethics (2008). Retrieved October 24, 2009 from Hospital Authority Head Office, Clinical Effectiveness & Technology Management Department, Web site: http://www.ha.org.hk/ho/research_ethics/rec_home.htm.

Kay, C. D. (1997). *Notes on DEONTOLOGY.* Retrieved October 20, 2009 from Wofford College, Department of Philosophy Web site: http://webs.wofford.edu/kaycd/ethics/deon.htm.

Moss, J. (2005). *Writing Clinical Research Protocols: Ethical Considerations.* Bulington: Academic Press, p. 3-4.

Moule, P. & Goodman, M. (2009). *Nursing Research: An Introduction.* London: SAGE Publications Ltd.

Newall, P. (2005). *Introducing Philosophy 11: Ethics.* Retrieved November 25, 2009 from The Galilean Library, Web site: http://www.galilean-library.org/manuscript.php?postid=43789.

Polit, D. F. & Beck, C. T. (2008). *Nursing research: generating and assessing evidence for nursing practice.* Philadelphia: Wolters Kluwer Health/Lippincott Williams & Wilkins.

Polit, D. F. & Beck, C. T. (2004). *Nursing research: principles and methods, 7th edition.* Philadelphia: Lippincott Williams & Wilkins.

Portney, L. G., & Watkins, M. P., (2009). *Foundations of clinical research: applications to practice.* Upper Saddle River: Pearson/Prentice Hall.

Ryan, K. J., Brady, J. V. & Cooke, R. E. (1979). *The Belmont Report, Office of the Secretary, Ethical Principles and Guidelines for the Protection of Human Subjects of Research, The National Commission for the Protection of Human Subjects of Biomedical and Behavioral Research.* Retrieved November 19, 2009 from U.S. Health & Human Services, Department of Health, Education, and Welfare, Web site: http://www.hhs.gov/ohrp/humansubjects/guidance/belmont.htm.

Tadd, W. (2003). *Ethics in nursing education, research and management: perspectives from Europe.* Basingstoke: Palgrave Macmillan.

In: Clinical Research Issues in Nursing     ISBN: 978-1-61668-937-7
Editor: Z. C. Y. Chan, pp.151-159    © 2010 Nova Science Publishers, Inc.

*Chapter XIV*

# Clinical Research Ethics

## *C. S. Fong and Zenobia C. Y. Chan*
The Hong Kong Polytechnic University, China

## Abstract

Clinical research plays an important role for building up knowledge and evidence base for nursing practices. It is important to maintain the accuracy of clinical research findings. Humans are the common interest in clinical research; it includes vulnerable groups like children, elderly and pregnant women. However, almost all research involving human beings is intrusive, as participants' information and feelings, which might otherwise be entirely personal, need to be published in research report. Thus, ethics are essential in clinical research to protect participants and to ensure the veracity of the research findings. Principles of research ethics provide a framework for researchers to maintain a common standard of clinical research conduct.

## Introduction

Research is becoming more important in nursing stream, which promotes evidence-based practices. Evidence-based practice depends on the research findings. The common participants for nursing research are usually related to patients, especially the vulnerable population with actual or potential health impairments such as the children, elderly and mentally ill. Researches involving humans are always with a certain degree of intrusion. Data collected in the research has to be elicited, but the data may be very private to the participants. Therefore, guidelines are needed for protecting the participants. Also, since the purpose of research is to build up a scientific foundation and theories for improvement of nursing practice, the veracity of the research data and results are crucial, otherwise the false research data can lead to improper nursing practices that can be harmful to the health system.

The objective of this chapter is to investigate the issue in clinical nursing ethics. Firstly to clarify the definition of research ethics in nursing, then to proceed to the principles and strategies to maintain the clinical research conduct.

## Meanings of Clinical Ethics

From the definitions in *The New Oxford American Dictionary*, ethics is the study of moral principles (2005, p.578). It concerns the goodness and badness of human behavior, or the principles of conduct related to right and wrong. Beauchamp and Childress (2001) describe the morality as the stable social consensus on the norms about right and wrong human conduct. Ethics in clinical research is the widely accepted standard of conduct related to clinical research. Nursing profession has code of conduct, guiding nurses in protecting patients. Ethical principles in clinical research are the guidelines for nurse researchers to protect the participants in research, also to ensure the truth of the research data. There are some international codes of conduct, for example, the *Code of Ethics for Nurses* (2006), produced by International Council of Nurses; *Nuremberg Code* (1947), the *Helsinki Declaration* (1964) and the *Data Protection Acts* (2003). In response to the above, *Data Protection Acts* (2003) provides the most applicable guidelines on protection of personal data of clinical research participants.

## Importance of Clinical Ethics

Scientific research is the basis for the development of professional nursing disciplines, to ensure the delivery of quality and cost-effective nursing service to the society. In the *Research strategy for nursing and midwifery in Ireland* (2003), nursing research is defined as:

> The process of answering questions and/or exploring phenomena using scientific methods; these methods may draw on the whole spectrum of systematic and critical inquiry (p.16).

The ultimate goal of nursing research is to develop an organized body of scientific knowledge through purposeful and systematic collection, analysis and interpretation of data. Nursing is a practice discipline; developing knowledge is crucial to guide practice and to improve the health and well-being of clients (Polit & Beck, 2004). Since research findings are to reflect and solve problems of the present phenomena in nursing discipline, the veracity of findings in nursing research is important to guide practice to maintain nursing care as evidence-based. The data collection and analysis should avoid bias, and the research results should be truthful and reflect the facts, otherwise, negative impacts may be brought to the health care system.

Moreover, some research participants may not be able to fully understand the harm brought by the research and thus are unable to make consent or are unable to withhold consent if they are put under implicit or explicit pressure (Moule & Goodman, 2009). Research ethics plays a key role to protect this vulnerable group. Furthermore, Moule & Goodman (2009) pointed out that when nurses act as a researcher in clinical setting, nurses have a dual role of researcher and care provider. Nurses themselves may face the possible conflict between duty to care and duty to advocate knowledge (Smith, 1997). Patients can be easily coerced or misled to participate in research project by wrongly assuming that it is a part of their nursing care. Participants who see researchers as nurses may be exploited and disclose too much. Therefore, a set of clear rules for clinical research ethics is important to protect both the nursing professional development and study participants.

# Principles of Clinical Research Ethics

Ethical principles act as a framework in guiding the researcher through the research process and its subsequent use. These principles must be adhered to by nurses to make sure every aspect of research is of the highest possible standard. The ethical principles have been mentioned by many authors in the literature; the common principles for nursing research are veracity, justice, non-malfeasance, beneficence, confidentiality and respect for persons (Beauchamp & Childress, 2001; Polit & Beck, 2004; Storch et al., 2004).

From the perspective of protecting participants, principle of veracity, non-malfeasance, confidentiality and respect are the essential components. Veracity is about reflecting the truth, related to the trusting relationship with participants (Pilot & Beck, 2004). Researchers should inform participants of all the potential risks and benefits if they take part in the research. Participants have the autonomy to choose participating or not and the flexibility to withdraw at any time without any coercion. We agree that potential participants should be notified about the amount or time and contribution they are expected to give and the gain and loss at the beginning so that they can decide voluntarily. Non-malfeasance is the duty to do no harm to research participants (Pilot & Beck, 2004). The harm should be avoided from all aspects including physical, mental, emotional, and socio-economical aspects. Special attention should to be placed on the vulnerable groups who cannot protect themselves.

Confidentiality is to keep the personal information that was collected from the study safe (Pilot & Beck, 2004). The access of this data is only permissible with participants' permission. Researchers have a responsibility to store the data in a safe place. Confidentiality not only can give protection to participants but also give participants a secure feeling. This improves the willingness of participants to take part in and give more information in the study. For that reason, we agree that promise to keep the personal data safe and undisclosed should be ensured to participants. Respect for persons includes respecting people's autonomy, their right to choose freely for themselves (Gillis and Jackson, 2002). In order to make autonomous decision, it needs informed choice. We believe that participants should be given sufficient information like the potential risks and benefits if participate in study, to understand the implications from the choice they make. Apart from protecting participants, veracity and beneficial nature are vital in a clinical research. Principle of Justice and beneficence give interpretation on this aspect. Justice is about the matter of fairness (Pilot & Beck, 2004). Different participants are being treated equally, without any discrimination over others. Random selection of participants can avoid unfairness in sample selection. Distribution of risks and benefits can be based on the participant's efforts, needs and rights. Beneficence is the duty to do good to both research participants and society (Pilot & Beck, 2004). The research is expected to benefit both the individual participants and society in general. One of the nurse's roles is client advocate;

if research interventions do more harm than benefit to study participants, nursing intervention is needed.

These are the basic principles of the clinical research ethics. Different research designs will need to have their specific ethical considerations to ensure the research evidence is produced ethically whilst employing good research practices. For example, in some ethnographic studies such as observation of behavior of a community, participants have no choice about participation, as they do not even know they are involved in the research.

# Strategies to Research Ethics

Some strategies can be applied to enact the above principles of the clinical research; they are informed consent, risk and benefit assessment, confidentiality procedures, debriefing and referral and external review.

Firstly, researchers are responsible to provide informed consent to participants. Informed consent refers to sufficient information provided to participants to decide whether to participate in the research. Researchers are responsible to inform participants about the study objective, expectation on participants' contribution like the time required, the voluntary nature of participation and the possible risk and benefits. A consent form is provided to participants, to serve as a proof that participants fully understand the research project and are willing to be involved in it. The Nuremberg Code defines informed consent (1947) as:

> The voluntary consent of the human subject is absolutely essential. This means that the person involved should have legal capacity to give consent; should be so situated as to be able to exercise free power of choice, without the intervention of any element of force, fraud, deceit, duress, over-reaching or other ulterior form of constraint or coercion; and should have sufficient knowledge and comprehension of the elements of the subject matter involved as to enable him to make an understanding and enlightened decision (Boomgaarden 2003 et al., p.108).

Although this definition is from an old article from 1947, the key points of the informed consent are still relevant nowadays. Participants should be provided sufficient information about the research project in order to allow them to make consent on the study. Beauchamp and Childress (2001) identified four essential components required for a valid informed consent: disclosure of information, comprehension, competency and voluntariness.

Therefore, when these four essential components are fulfilled in the informed consent, we can ensure participant fully understand the study and is willing to be involved voluntarily.

Secondly, risk-benefit assessments should be performed prior to the collection of data. Balance between potential benefits and risk on participants and society should be achieved. The benefit and risk to research participants includes physical, like being involved in a potentially beneficial treatment that otherwise would not be accessible to them and unanticipated side effects of the testing treatment—emotional, like having a friendly and objective researcher to discuss participant's problem in a comfortable way and the psychological distress as a result of self-disclosure; and social, like loss of status and negative impact on personal relationship. The result of the research may benefit the whole society, however, the potential risk borne by participants should not overweigh the benefits of knowledge gain. The risk should be minimal. Polit and Beck (2010) defined minimal risk as the expected potential risk no greater than those ordinary risks experienced in daily life or during routine physical or psychological tests or procedures. Researchers should take caution to the risk and try to reduce the risk if it is unavoidable.

Thirdly, attention should be placed on confidentiality procedures. Researchers are responsible keeping the data provided by study participants in the strictest confidence. It can be carried out through anonymity. The confidentiality can be safeguarded, even if the researcher cannot identify the participants in their data. For example, distribute questionnaires without any identification information on the questionnaires and then responses would be anonymous. When collecting hospital records, all the identification information like name and address should be expunged. Anonymity can protect participant's right to privacy. If it is not feasible to keep anonymity, a promise of confidentiality should be performed. This is to ensure any information participants provided will be not be publicly reported in a manner that enables them to be identified. The confidentiality procedures of research data throughout the collection and analysis process can be performed by keeping identifying information in locked files to limit accessibility, to use identification numbers to replace participants' names on data records, and to only report the aggregate data for groups of participants or to take steps to mask a person's identity in a research report. If it is a qualitative study that includes only few participants, substituting a fictitious name and not showing the information like age and occupation that can reflect the characteristics of participants is important to protect the confidence of the informants.

In addition, debriefing and referral can be carried out to care for the emotional risk and show respect to study participants proactively. It can be done through carefully attending to the nature of the interactions they have with the participants. The researchers should be gentle and polite, use wordings tactfully, and be sensitive to cultural differences. To show respect to participants, researchers can give participants the study findings after the data analysis process. A formal debriefing can be offered after the completion of data collection, to let participants to raise questions and complaints. If stress is produced throughout the data collection process or the deception has been made on the ethical guidelines, it is particularly important to hold a debriefing to clarify. If the participants' emotional problems cannot be solved in the debriefing, researchers may need to help by making referrals for participants to appropriate health, social and psychological services.

Besides, external review is important to exclude bias and ensure the fulfillment of the clinical research ethics. Researchers may have difficulty being completely objective when performing the risk-benefit assessments or when setting up procedures to protect participants' benefit. Scope and level of knowledge, desire to conduct a valid study can cause biases. In order to minimize bias, the ethical dimensions of a study are usually sent for an external review. The external reviewer may be the committees set up in hospitals, universities or other institutions for reviewing research plans. Getting ethical review and approval is the first important step to conducting a research.

# Research Misconduct

Some common misconduct in research should be avoided. It includes fabrication, falsification and plagiarism. Fabrication involves making up data or study results. Falsification is the manipulation of research materials, equipment, or processes and also the change and omission of data or distortion of results (Pilot & Beck, 2004). These lead to an inaccurate report. Plagiarism refers to taking credit for someone's ideas, results, or words inappropriately, or without providing credit. We consider that insisting on the veracity of data and results is one of the critical principles of research. Giving correct credit to references is also essential to show respect to the authors.

# Conclusion

Nursing research involves human participants and usually takes participants who are unable to protect themselves. Findings of research provide knowledge and evidence support to the nursing development. Thus, protecting participants and ensuring the truth of research findings are important issues in clinical research ethics. Honesty, openness, respect and sensitivity to participants are the top priorities in clinical research ethics. To safeguard the benefits and minimize risks, it is important that all nursing research following clear ethical principles and guidelines. Ethical concerns should be taken into consideration at the beginning of a research problem, maintaining all over the whole process of data collection, analysis and report. Researchers' perspectives on ethical principles and external committee review provide double safeguards to the research conduct.

# Author's Background

Fong Chi Sum is a student of Master of Nursing programme in The Hong Kong Polytechnic University. Her research interest is on the positive working environment for nurses. (Email: tracy_fg@yahoo.com.hk)

# References

An Bord Altranais. (2007). Guidance to nurses and midwives regarding ethical conduct of nursing and midwifery research. An Bord Altranais.

Beauchamp, T.L. and Childress, J. F. (2001). Principles of biomedical ethics. Oxford: Oxford University Press.

Boomgaarden J., Louhiala P. and Wiesing U. (2003). Issues in Medical Research Ethics—A Workbook for Practitioners and Students. New York: Berghahn Books.

Department of Health and Children (2003). Research strategy for nursing and midwifery in Ireland. Dublin: The Stationery Office.

Gillis, A and Jackson, W. (2002). Research for nurses: methods and interpretation. Philadelphia: F.A. Davis Co.

International Council of Nurses (1996). Ethical guidelines for nursing research. Geneva: International Council of Nurses.

McKean, E. (2005). The new Oxford American dictionary. New York; Oxford University Press.

Moule, P. & Goodman, M. (2009). *Nursing research: an introduction.* London: Thousand Oaks.

Polit, D. F. & Beck, C. T. (2010). *Essentials of nursing research: appraising evidence for nursing practice.* Philadelphia: Wolters Kluwer Health/Lippincott Williams & Wilkins.

Polit D. F. & Beck C. T. (2004). Nursing research: principles and methods. 7th ed. Philadelphia: Lippincott, Williams and Wilkins.

Smith, P. (1997). Research mindedness for practice: an interactive approach for nursing and health care. New York: Churchill Livingstone.

Storch J., Rodney P. & Starzomski R. (2004). Towards a moral horizon: nursing ethics for leadership and practice. Canada: Pearson Prentice Hall.

# Index